THE
HOT
GUIDE
TO A
COOL
Sexy
MENOPAUSE

Nurse Barb's
Practical Advice
& Real-Life Solutions
for a Smooth
Transition

THE
HOT
GUIDE
TO A
COOL
Sexy
MENOPAUSE

BARBARA DEHN R.N., M.S., N.P.

Basic Health
PUBLICATIONS, INC.

The information contained in this book is based upon the research and personal and professional experiences of the author. It is not intended as a substitute for consulting with your physician or other healthcare provider. Any attempt to diagnose and treat an illness should be done under the direction of a healthcare professional.

The publisher does not advocate the use of any particular healthcare protocol but believes the information in this book should be available to the public. The publisher and author are not responsible for any adverse effects or consequences resulting from the use of the suggestions, preparations, or procedures discussed in this book. Should the reader have any questions concerning the appropriateness of any procedures or preparation mentioned, the author and the publisher strongly suggest consulting a pro-fessional healthcare advisor.

Basic Health Publications, Inc.
28812 Top of the World Drive
Laguna Beach, CA 92651
949-715-7327 • www.basichealthpub.com

Library of Congress Cataloging-in-Publication Data

Dehn, Barbara
  The hot guide to a cool, sexy menopause : nurse Barb's practical advice and
real-life solutions for a smooth transition / Barbara Dehn, R.N., M.S., N.P.
     pages cm
   Includes bibliographical references and index.
   ISBN 978-1-59120-371-1
   1. Menopause—Popular works. I. Title.
   RG186.D44   2014
   618.1'75—dc23

                                                           2014009344

Editor: Carol Killman Rosenberg • www.carolkillmanrosenberg.com
Typesetting/Book design: Gary A. Rosenberg • www.thebookcouple.com
Cover design: Jan Davis • www.JanDavisDesign.com

Printed in the United States of America

10   9   8   7   6   5   4   3   2   1

Contents

Acknowledgments

$\mathcal{T}$his book is a result of years of listening to friends and patients describe how their lives were turned upside down by the hormonal roller coaster of menopause and how much they wanted their lives back. Then, when I began feeling the fire of hot flashes and couldn't sleep more than a few hours without throwing off the covers and leaping out of bed to douse myself with cold water, I really understood how completely menopause can alter a woman's life. I wasn't ready to throw in the towel, and I knew that millions of women weren't either.

I'm especially grateful to all of the women who graciously shared their experiences with me and provided the stories in each chapter. Their honesty and desire to find options to relieve their symptoms provided the genesis of this book. I'm deeply grateful to my colleagues at Women Physicians Medical Group in Mountain View, California, for inspiring and modeling how to partner with patients. Dr. Katherine Sutherland, Dr. Christine Litwin-Sanguinetti, Dr. Janet Pulskamp, and Dr. Rita Leard, I learned so much from each of you about how to be a better clinician and listener. I'm also deeply grateful to the friends who generously agreed to review multiple drafts of this manuscript, cover options, make spot-on suggestions, and provide constant support and encouragement along the way: Marilyn Arnst, Carol Weiss, Mary Dean, Therese McKenna, Kathy Augason, Karen Avery, Beth Dawes, Leslie Pinkelman, Lauren Zucchi, Susan Alfano, Margaret Braccio, Cathy Konicki, Judi Rich, Alison Takata, Sidney Johnson, Claudia Winkelman, Teri Zingale, my friends from the 100 Women Foundation and the friends who meet for coffee, hikes, and Homestead band events.

I am especially grateful to my nurse practitioner colleagues: Mimi Secor, Diane Todd-Pace, Lisa Chism, Deb Kiley, Nancy Dirubbo, Karen Ketner, Jenny Shipp, and Mary Foehringer. I'd also like to thank my colleagues at the North American Menopause Society for providing evidence-based resources for women at midlife.

I'm deeply indebted to Jan Davis, who designed the cover of this book and who has been the designer for my Personal Guides to Health. I'd also like to thank my fantastic team at Media 2x3, Adora English, and Jess Ponce, who believed in the importance of empowering women with information and encouraged me to write this book.

This book benefited from the insight and coaching of Dr. Joyce Starr and from my energetic and engaging agent, Karen Gantz Zahler. I'd also like to thank Norman Goldfind, an extraordinary publisher who loved the title and his outstanding team at Basic Health Publishing, especially Carol Killman Rosenberg, who edited the manuscript.

I am also grateful to my parents and especially to my son, Giancarlo. His sense of humor and patience with a mom who talks about hot flashes and menopause makes me so proud of the wonderful man he's becoming.

And most of all, I am lucky to have a cool sexy menopause because of my best friend and the love of my life: my husband, John. His patience, support, wisdom, and encouragement mean everything to me. I am deeply grateful.

Introduction

Menopause can impact a woman's life in a variety of ways. The range of experiences is as varied and unique as each woman's own life. For some women, menopause feels like a mild breeze, bringing few concerns and only minor physical changes. For other women, it feels like they are being challenged by a Category-5 hurricane that wreaks havoc in every aspect of their lives. For the rest, the experience of menopause falls somewhere in the middle.

Whatever the case may be, my patients and friends who are experiencing menopausal symptoms aren't ready to just accept whatever "weather" comes their way. We aren't our grandmothers' generation! We want to maintain our vitality and zest—and yes, our sexy outlook—during this stage of our lives.

The Hot Guide to a Cool Sexy Menopause is an extension of what I offer my patients, which is to provide relatable information, explanations, and a menu of options to consider. I don't believe in telling women what to do when they are challenged by the hormonal roller-coaster ride that comes with menopause. Instead, I believe that each woman needs to find her own best path and try various solutions, as she makes the wisest and healthiest choices in her own life.

No matter what your personal experience has been with menopause so far, it is likely you have some bothersome symptoms and many questions. This book offers vital information, answers, practical tips, and a few secrets that have helped thousands of women stride confidently through this transition with more health, vitality, and even more sexiness than ever before.

Menopause isn't the end, nor is it something to be endured like a root canal. Menopause is a new beginning and can be one of the most rewarding times in your life. There's a great deal to look forward to during this part of your journey and beyond. For many women, menopause may be the first time in their lives that they fully give themselves permission to do what they want, rather than what is expected of them. Many women find newfound freedom to explore new opportunities or to devote more time to the activities that nurture and sustain them. As their bodies change, many women find themselves restless and ready to reexamine their lives and redirect their path toward new destinations.

By the time you've reached this stage of your life, there's a good chance you feel more alive and more energized than ever before. You're smarter, wiser, and more in touch with yourself than you were ten or twenty years ago, and yet you may still feel sideswiped by the physical changes your body is undergoing and how you're feeling. Some or much of what you're experiencing might even be overwhelming or confusing. My job is to help you make sense of what you're facing and serve up some practical advice, experience, humor, and research-based solutions that have helped millions of menopausal women feel their best. Each chapter covers a different aspect of the menopause transition. For each topic, I'll also share real women's experiences with the physical, emotional, and spiritual challenges of menopause and describe how they navigated this journey, growing stronger, more empowered, and healthier. The "Nitty-Gritty" sections cover all the basics you need to know, and each chapter ends with my hot tips and secrets that will give you the edge over each menopausal challenge.

After caring for women for over twenty-five years, I know that every woman is different and wants advice tailored to her own unique life and situation, with options to choose from that will be the best for her. I know the same is true for you. Enjoy your journey.

1

Letting Go and Reclaiming Your Life

I have some good news and some bad news. The bad news is that menopause usually sneaks up on us at midlife when our plates are already overflowing with the responsibilities of work, family, aging parents, and to-do lists that seem to get longer every day. The last thing we need is the unpredictability of menopause with sleep deprivation, hot flashes, night sweats, or other physical and emotional challenges. The good news is that menopause arrives at midlife at a time when most women have the skills they need to deal with whatever comes their way.

By the time our periods stop all together, we're much more likely to be very comfortable in our own skin—more than we ever felt before. When menopausal symptoms such as hot flashes and night sweats begin to appear, it's likely that we finally have the wisdom, the time, and the moxie to listen to our hearts and forge ahead on our own paths. It's an empowering and uplifting time, and most of the time we feel great. However, even the most self-confident among us have minutes or even days when we look in the mirror and wish that the woman with a few wrinkles and gray roots who's staring back was more reflective of how young and vibrant we feel on the inside.

The good news is that you've learned and experienced a lot in the last forty or fifty years, which will help you successfully navigate this next part of your journey. At midlife and menopause, our bodies are experiencing profound physical changes that can spark profound emotional, personal,

3

and spiritual transformations. With bodies, minds, and spirits so intimately interconnected, menopause offers an opportunity for a renaissance of sorts with a renewed drive toward more creative, spiritual, and professional fulfillment. Many of my patients have described "waking up" and feeling somewhat the same and yet so different that they've been driven to reexamine their lives and chart new paths toward the lives they want. What's amazing to me is that all of these inner transformations are occurring during a period of intense physical change, which makes it all the more impressive.

Let me introduce you to three women—Jackie, Tina, and Maggie—whose emotional lives may seem very familiar to you. You may even recognize yourself in one or more of them.

JACKIE'S STORY

Jackie was in a quandary. She needed to get to her meeting on time, but her blouse was already soaked and it had only been ten minutes since she put it on. She was already running late from waiting until her hot flashes eased up enough to put on her makeup. She had precious little patience available to deal with anything that wasn't an emergency. Her phone was vibrating and the caller ID revealed an old friend who was driving her nuts. "Oh, jeez," she groaned. "If I pick it up, I'll be on the phone for a half hour listening to the laundry list of things wrong with her life. Ugh." The last thing Jackie wanted to do right now was take care of someone else, especially this friend who seemed to suck all of her energy into a black hole of negativity.

Jackie didn't want to enter the Dark Side, where this particular friend seemed to spend most of her time. Though Jackie was known by most of her friends as Mrs. McNice, because she always put others first, right now was not the best time to be a supportive listener. This friend was always complaining about the most insignificant things imaginable. Jackie felt used. As tired and wrung out as she felt with her own drenching and frequent hot flashes, there were far worse things that people were dealing with. The one good thing about menopause, with its debilitating hot flashes, night sweats, and sleep deprivation, was that her patience had worn wafer thin, and she had very little time to listen to whining. She no longer had the energy to be Mrs. McNice all the time.

Jackie felt as if she were stepping into a steam room multiple times throughout the day and had to dash off to the bathroom to run cold water over her wrists. These frequent trips gave her more time to think about the people and situations that were dragging her down.

Jackie let the call roll over to voice mail and felt instantly gratified. She also felt slightly surprised by her lack of guilt. Of course the stress of making that decision had brought about yet another hot flash, but it was worth it, she reasoned, as she took some slow deep breaths to let it pass and then went to find a dry blouse. Not picking up the phone and deciding to ignore her misplaced sense of obligation made her feel so much lighter. She smiled, knowing that she was making the decision to put her own needs first, at least for the next half hour.

Jackie's menopause brought insistent hot flashes and night sweats, demanding instant cooling measures and a breath of fresh air. She was beginning to think that some aspects of her life could also use freshening, like this particularly negative friend and a coworker who wasn't delivering, to name a few. Lately, Jackie felt that there was so little time left in each day that she couldn't afford to waste it on people or activities that suffocated her optimism and left her feeling drained. The hot flashes were draining most of her energy, and she didn't have much left to spare for people who were making it worse.

Over the last few months, Jackie noticed her exhaustion and irritability increasing as her hot flashes increased. Before she had to adapt to the challenges of menopause, Jackie had been putting up with exasperating people and situations, not wanting to make waves. Lately, however, she found that she was unapologetically speaking her mind more directly and not sugarcoating everything so that everyone would like her. Exhaustion had wiped the guilt slate clean, and, frankly, she felt more freedom to be herself, speak up, and not try to be Mrs. McNice all the time just to keep the peace. To her surprise, she also found that being more direct and not caring as much about what others thought didn't cause the upset she always strived to avoid. Amazingly, people could actually handle the truth. Jackie resolved not to avoid this friend the next time she called, but to suggest instead that her friend see a therapist.

When Jackie came to see me to discuss remedies for her hot flashes, she also wanted to talk about how menopause had changed her way of dealing with the world—in positive ways. A friend had changed her nickname from Mrs. McNice to Mrs. McFierce one day when she calmly and confidently confronted an irritating clerk. The nickname had stuck, and we laughed about Jackie tapping into her inner fierce and ferocious tiger when necessary. Instead of being put off by her strength, Jackie found that her friends and coworkers welcomed it when they themselves were also in similar situations. She found herself being more comfortable saying, "No," and "No, thank you," to people and situations that in the past she had invariably said, "Yes" to, only to feel resentful about the time and energy wasted on things she really didn't want to do. There was a shift now in how she handled work situations, friends, family, other parents at her kids' schools, and even her husband. What was even more empowering was that Jackie knew in her heart that there was no turning back to the old, accommodating ways. The freedom she now felt to speak up and speak out had been triggered by her lack of sleep, but as she felt better physically and had more restful nights, she found that she was much happier being honest with others and standing up for herself. She didn't have to be a doormat or strive to always be nice to a fault; tapping into her fierce inner tiger when the situation called for it also helped her feel more authentic.

TINA'S DILEMMA

Experiencing menopausal symptoms is often the wake-up call that helps women begin to reexamine where they are on their own priority list. The best multitasker in the book club, Tina's plate wasn't just full, it was overflowing. The trouble was, she told herself, if you want something done right, you should just do it yourself. And what's more, she knew that she could finish something in the time it took to explain how to do it to someone else. Even with a demanding full-time job that included traveling coast to coast twice each month, a husband and two teenagers and helping to care for her elderly mom, Tina was still able to throw an impromptu dinner party without breaking a sweat. She never complained, was always smiling, and was so well organized that things just ran smoothly.

Then Tina's life suddenly turned upside down. Overnight, she felt completely different and out of control. She started waking up drenched in sweat four to eight times each night. Getting back to sleep seemed to take hours, and just as she'd drift off in an exhausted state, another drenching night sweat would come on with an insistent sensation that her bladder was full, yet again. Tina could no longer keep up her incredibly busy, highly efficient pace. Flying red-eyes across the country, which were no big deal in the past, were now impossible. She was beyond irritable. Tina's typically warm smile faded into a cold grimace. Tina felt too young for night sweats and menopause, and yet they arrived without warning, like an audit notice from the Internal Revenue Service. Oh no, not this, not now!

Tina had been sailing along, doing everything for everyone and accomplishing more in a day than most people do in a month. During one of her restless nights brought on by wave after wave of night sweats, Tina thought about all the little and big things she wasn't getting around to because of her crushing exhaustion. She also wrestled with the feeling that all of her time was eaten up doing the things she felt compelled to complete and guilty about if she didn't, so that there was no time left to do what she wanted to do.

One weekend morning, her daughter suggested that they go to a local yoga studio. Tina gritted her teeth and felt like snapping, "I don't have time to go to yoga. Have you taken a look around this house? And what about Grandma?" but instead she took a deep breath and shrugged her shoulders. She heard that yoga was supposed to be good for you. Since she also wanted to spend some time with her daughter, Tina grudgingly relented and went along to a beginner's class. She felt so much better afterward. It was hard to explain, she told me, but going to her daughter's yoga class felt like she had turned an important corner in her life.

Soon, Tina was going to a yoga class with her daughter or a friend one to two times each week. Holding the positions was a challenge she enjoyed, but the quiet meditation at the end was such an unexpected source of calm that she found herself returning to the yoga studio regularly. She was surprised that for once she was actually carving out some time for her own needs. Tina wasn't sure if it was her weekly commitment to yoga or if it was her commitment to doing something just for herself that recharged her energy and enthusiasm. As she pondered that question one week while lying in a relaxed pose, she realized that it really didn't matter. She was finally allowing herself the space and time to let go of things she had to do, which freed up energy for what she wanted to do.

Reading the assigned book for her book club was one of the first casualties of letting go of the "I shoulds." Tina recognized that showing up to socialize without having read that month's selection was a very small step in putting herself first, and yet it felt like a gigantic leap toward more control of her life.

As Tina worked on managing her night sweats, she also worked on managing how she wanted to live her life. She told me that her life used to be a series of events that she would make happen, get through, and then start planning for whatever was next on the list. "I wasn't really there completely," she explained. "I was always thinking about the details, what people might be thinking, and if everything was exactly the way I planned. I realized that I was never really 100 percent fully immersed in any of those activities. I was always thinking about all the things I needed to do and then what the next item on the list would entail."

Because she was so organized and could do a million and one things, Tina felt like an event planner, not someone who enjoyed all the trouble she went through. Once the night sweats rocked Tina's world and her sleep changed, she used it as an opportunity to really look at her life and what made her happy. Tina still travels, but now she's making time not just for work conferences but also for yoga retreats. She still throws a great dinner party, but instead of running around making sure everyone's glass is full, she's sitting down, talking, and laughing. Everyone's having lots more fun because she's having lots more fun, not sweating the details.

MAGGIE'S STORY

Before menopause rolled into her life, Maggie would never have considered starting her own business as a caterer. For the last twenty-five years, all of her focus and all of her time was devoted to her family, and, as is the case with virtually every woman with a family they came first. Her days were packed with volunteering at various schools, shuttling kids from one activity to the next, and making sure everyone had exactly what they needed at all times. She was exhausted by the end of the day and yet there was something missing. She couldn't quite put her finger on what it was, but she had the sense that her life was really not hers at all. Her life was defined by everyone else's expectations and these drove her daily routine as the years marched on. She wasn't happy with the status quo, but wasn't sure she could make the leap to something completely different.

Maggie was enormously proud of her kids and loved her life, but as she started noticing more and more of the physical changes from menopause, she had the sense that time was not infinite. She couldn't quite shake the nagging whisper in her ear that there was a lot more out there than just waiting to be a grandmother. As one child after another left the nest and needed her less and less, she started to wonder what she was going to do with all of her time. More important, she began to think about not just filling up her time, but looking for something she could feel excited about. Maggie loved to cook. Poring over cookbooks was one of her favorite ways to relax and unwind. She also enjoyed having people over because that meant she could try out new recipes. She often wondered what it would be like to become a caterer.

Maggie had to admit that she was more than a little overwhelmed at the thought of starting a business from scratch. How would she finance it? How would she advertise, get clients, set prices, and deliver the food? She made lists in her head of all the things that could go wrong. She wanted to do it, but it seemed daunting.

Maggie came to see me for an embarrassing concern related to menopause. In addition to needing to wear a pad to soak up leaking urine, she was also thirty pounds overweight and her elevated blood sugar levels put her at risk for diabetes. As we worked together on helping her lose weight and get her blood sugar to a healthy level, I also suggested that she start pelvic-floor-strengthening classes. After seeing that just two classes helped reduce her leaking, Maggie's motivation to lose weight soared. Within months, her bladder was behaving itself and she had lost twelve pounds. Now, instead of simply shrugging and accepting whatever life threw her way, Maggie was taking charge of her life. She set realistic goals and found that they weren't as difficult as she had imagined.

As Maggie took charge of the physical aspects of her life, she began to feel more confident. "If I can lose twelve pounds and not have to wear *adult diapers," she reasoned, "I can do anything." As she talked to herself, she realized that she had been overwhelmed by the enormity of starting a business, and instead she could take baby steps first. She decided that working for a caterer was a good way to dip her toe into the water before diving in headfirst.*

THE NITTY-GRITTY ON LETTING GO

As estrogen levels wane in menopause, our brain chemistry alters. Some neurobiologists believe that the drop in estrogen manifests with more indifference to what men think about us. Unlike adolescence, with surging levels of estrogen bathing our brains in a hormonal soup that drove us toward a complete obsession with how we looked and what others thought, menopause does the opposite. In menopause, women frankly don't give a damn about trying to please men or be the most attractive female in the room. This may also partly explain how less competition for men results in deepening female friendships at this stage of life.

During menopause, we also come to grips with the very real fact that our bodies are finished having babies. The life-giving part of our life is over, unless we decide to spend thousands of dollars and use donor eggs. I know that this can be very difficult. Some women need to grieve the loss of their fertility and their ability to become pregnant. Others are happy to finish that chapter. Those doors are closing and the numerous physical changes in menopause remind us that our lives really are different than they used to be. One look in the magnifying mirror is often all it takes to see the evidence staring back at us. We're not the dewy-faced, inexperienced girl we used to be.

No Time to Waste

Menopause offers an opportunity to remind us of our own mortality. As we confront the fact that the time we have left is not infinite, we're less and less likely to squander that time on pursuits that have lost their meaning. What impresses me about women at menopause is that many make the choice not to be depressed or defeated by the idea of a finite amount of time left, but to be energized and excited about what's to come. The old clichés apply at menopause. It's almost as if we receive a reminder that life is not a "dress rehearsal," "the clock is ticking," and there's "no time like the present." It's high time to live our own dreams.

New Paths to Take

As we watch our ability to get pregnant fade in the rearview mirror, what lies ahead are many other options to generate, sustain, and nurture life. As the exhausting daily work of bearing and raising children occupies less of our energy, there's one person who can finally take center stage. You're wondering who that is, aren't you? No, it's not your kids or your partner, your parents, your pets, your friends, or your coworkers. It's not the organizations you generously volunteer your time to. It's someone very close to you. Give up? That person is YOU!

I've seen women move from caring for their family 24/7 to starting nonprofits that care for people around the world. I have patients who've gone back to school to be architects, therapists, and pastry chefs. I know women who decided that they'd really rather sell houses and others who are writing novels and blogs. I know women who've entered politics and others who are building schools in Africa. At menopause and beyond, there's a tremendous surge of energy and a desire to look for new life-giving, generative directions and outlets for our nurturing spirits.

Saying "No" So That You Can Say "Yes"

Learning how to say, "No" or "No, thank you," is another huge milestone for most of us at menopause. It may not be a challenge for our daughters, but for most of us who were raised to put others first, saying no can be a daunting task. Prior to dealing with debilitating hot flashes and night sweats that sapped our energy, we could say "Yes" to everything, turning ourselves into pretzels to make everything work for everyone else.

Before menopause steals into our lives, we're ultimate multitaskers, which is good up to a point. But when is enough, enough? For many of my patients, menopause changes everything. When hot flashes and night sweats start and a good night's sleep becomes a rare and precious thing, many of us suddenly become more likely to bite someone's head off. Let's face it, when you're sleep deprived, being polite isn't a high priority. You're just trying to survive and get through the day so that you can climb back into bed and pray for a few hours of precious, don't-bother-me, leave-me-alone, cherished, uninterrupted sleep.

Learning how to begin taking care of yourself may be as simple as learning a new communication technique. There's a skill to saying "No" or "I wish I could, but I can't." These are polite and also wonderful ways that help you take care of your own needs.

When you're dealing with night sweat–induced sleep deprivation, suddenly, "good" becomes "good enough." At this point, we don't feel the need to go that extra mile, because our experience tells us that we can get the same results with less effort. We're not as keen on trying to keep up with or impress others, because by now we're much more comfortable with ourselves. We know we have flaws and shortcomings, but who doesn't? It does take time to see that just as we accept others for who they are, our friends give that acceptance right back. We know that we don't have to be perfect to be worthy of love. We're beyond the giddiness of thinking that we need a certain house, specific pair of shoes, or box of dark chocolate to make us forever blissfully happy. We know that those things are nice and give flavor to our lives, but they don't define us; we define ourselves.

· ·

"I wish I could, but I can't."

I learned this great phrase working in my son's preschool. "I wish I could, but I can't." This simple phrase validates the request, grants the wish in fantasy, while also saying no gently. "Just say no" doesn't just apply to teens considering street drugs. It applies to every woman of menopausal age who raises her hand to volunteer to bake the cookies, bring the appetizer, drive the friend, host the party, raise the funds, fly to the meeting, or any of the other gazillion things we do every single day of every single week out of pure unadulterated obligation.

Don't get me wrong; women doing things out of obligation is how our communities stay knitted together and how all-volunteer organizations and nonprofits stay afloat. I'm not saying let it all go and spend your time indulging in manicures and pedicures, though at times that's tempting, isn't it? I am saying that what I've found for myself and for my patients is that finally, in menopause, it's so much easier to make yourself a priority. With sleep deprivation and the other physical changes, it's a welcome relief to let a few balls drop and to choose not to juggle so many all at once while balancing on one foot and eating an apple! Multitasking and being super-organized is way overrated. In menopause, it's much easier to walk toward more meaning in your life, not because you *have* to, but because you *want* to. There's a world of opportunity waiting when we let a few things drop and free ourselves from the "I shoulds."

In the stories I shared earlier, Maggie became more empowered and confident by overcoming her physical challenges, which led her to believe in more possibilities. Jackie and Tina took a different route toward empow-erment, but all three women made choices that were deeply rooted in what was best for them, not what was best for others.

. . . .

Put on Your Oxygen Mask First

In menopause, making your life, your dreams, and your health a priority will pay huge dividends now in how you feel day to day and later on in your long-term health and happiness. Your mood, your willingness to venture out to a larger world, and even your efficiency with the ever-expanding to-do list will all improve when you give yourself permission to prioritize your own happiness.

It is easy to feel overwhelmed by the idea of taking the first steps on a new path while tackling the physical and emotional challenges of menopause. However, if you lighten your load and shed some of the "I shoulds," you'll find a surprising surge of energy to confront other issues of concern. Just because you're strong enough to endure, doesn't mean you should. Think about what your life would look like if you could trans-fer the enormous amount of energy you expend daily on obligations and redirect it toward your own personal fulfillment. I guarantee you'll be amazed at what's possible. Not only will you have more energy, but you will also feel more confident, which translates into a much sexier and open outlook.

• •

Nurse Barb's Cool Menopause
Happiness & Fulfillment Tips

- **BREATHE DEEPLY**—Take ten deep breaths at least once day to help you find your calm, grounded center. As a bonus, this helps hot flashes, too.

- **MAKE TIME TO EXERCISE**—Thirty minutes each day will reduce your risk of diabetes and breast cancer and improve every aspect of your life, mood, health, and yes, even your sex drive.

- **NURTURE YOURSELF AS MUCH AS YOU NURTURE OTHERS**—Self-care is more important now than ever. No one can keep up a demanding pace without some time to recharge.

- **LIMIT LIVING IN THE PAST**—Acknowledge that you're different than you were twenty or thirty years ago. Take some time to grieve and then move on to your next chapter.

- **FLEX & STRETCH**—Stretching and flexibility training helps maintain the active lifestyle we all want and prevents injuries that can sideline us.

- **EXPLORE MORE**—Your brain is hungry for new experiences and thirsty for knowledge. Taking a class, learning a new skill, and traveling will nourish your brain and your spirit.

- **LOOK FOR MEANINGFUL OPPORTUNITIES**—There's never been a better time to share your gifts of wisdom, experience, and talent with the world. The possibilities are endless, with infinite opportunities for more fulfillment.

- **TAP INTO YOUR SILLINESS**—Laughter is your secret weapon, but so is whimsy and silliness and giggles. Now that you're free of the "I shoulds," it's the perfect time to step outside your comfort zone and have more fun.

- **GIRLFRIEND TIME**—Spending time with friends helps bathe our brains in feel-good chemicals, improves mood, and is the best therapy available.

- **CONSTRUCT CONFIDENCE**—Even if you're not completely there, stride into your confident zone, because there's nothing sexier than a confident woman.

• •

WHERE YOU'VE BEEN & WHERE YOU'RE GOING

In menopause, when you close the door on the "I shoulds" and begin to say, "No, thank you," new doors and new paths of possibility swing wide open. Your time is finite, and so is your energy. Menopause is an opportunity to reexamine where you've been and where you want to go.

Prior to menopause and midlife, many of us were good girls who always wanted to do the "right thing" all the time. What is the right thing though? Are we living our lives based on others' expectations of what we should be doing? Menopause is the perfect time to start considering the "what-ifs" and what's right for us

Menopause is a gift that provides the perfect opportunity to try on new roles. Do you want to teach a Zumba class? Start a new business? Write a novel? Travel the world? Channel your creativity? Run for office? Volunteer at a hospital? Chair a conference? Start a nonprofit? Create a garden? Change careers? Start a new relationship? Make new friends? Research your ancestors? Mentor someone? Take a class?

After all, with all of your rich life experience, you *can* do anything! First, it's important to shed the layers and layers of guilt, obligation, and the need to please so that you can listen to your own voice.

Ask yourself these two simple questions. First, "Does what I'm doing right now still have meaning for me?" and "Is this what I want to do for the next twenty to fifty years?"

Who knows what your journey looks like and where the paths you'll take will lead. No matter where you find yourself right now on the menopause map, making time for yourself, letting go of the "I shoulds," and being open to the "what-ifs" will all combine to increase your happiness, health, vitality, confidence, and your sexiness through menopause and beyond.

2

Making Peace or Declaring War on Your Skin

*S*eemingly overnight in menopause, we invariably wake up to a new reflection. The truth is, we don't look the way we did in our twenties and thirties. Thousands of women from around the country have told me the exact moment when they saw themselves as a mature woman and not a girl. Their reflection on the outside didn't sync with how they felt on the inside. When it comes to their skin around menopause, my patients are always asking me, "What happened?" As you'll read in this chapter, the hormonal changes of menopause influence how our skin looks and feels. It's not your imagination; your skin really is different now.

It can take minutes or months to grieve the loss of what was and then move on to acceptance, adaptation, or all-out war. With our society's emphasis on youth and beauty, women in menopause have a few more challenges than they did in their twenties. The good news is that by now, with your accumulated wisdom and experience, you'll be fine. Not only do you already have quite a few tricks up your sleeves, but I also have several secret weapons to share with you in this chapter.

The first secret is that tapping into a sexier menopause is all about our attitude, which comes from within, not from how we look on the outside. However, I know that looking our best helps us feel our best. As Billy Crystal, playing the character Fernando, used to say on *Saturday Night Live,* "It's better to look marvelous than to feel marvelous." This is funny, but it's not quite right for women in menopause. You see, one of our secret weapons is surprisingly simple: confidence. Regaining your confidence is the ultimate beauty treatment. Taking this quote and turning it upside down fits much better: "When you feel marvelous, you'll look marvelous!"

In menopause, feeling great on the inside boosts confidence. It creates an attractive inner glow, bringing out the twinkle and the spark, drawing people into our circles. Confident women are like attraction magnets; other people want to be around them—they're more vibrant, more enthusiastic, and everyone wants to shine in their light. They're sexier!

In menopause there's also a subtle, yet perceptible shift in a woman's perspective. This is another one of our secret weapons. We're well beyond caring too much about how we look and are more invested in what we think and how we feel. I've noticed that by the time a woman reaches menopause, she doesn't look exactly like all of her friends. This is very different from our twenties, when everyone had the same hairstyle, shoes, jeans, and jewelry. Now, with some life experience, we're less concerned about superficialities both in ourselves and in others. Of course, we want to look our best, but *being* ourselves is a powerful aphrodisiac.

Just as we look beneath the surface with others, by menopause we're not going to waste our time worrying about other people who judge "a book by its cover." We've accomplished so much in our lives that our validation comes from who we are and our contributions to our families, communities, and the world—not how we look. This shift in perspective is one of the most powerful secret weapons we have now.

Does it make sense to wear five-inch platform heels that crush the toes and are guaranteed to lead to an office visit with an orthopedic surgeon? Are you out of your mind? No way! Limping around in a cast may garner more sympathy, but it's not practical. In menopause, many women acquire the confidence to wear shoes that they could easily sprint in to catch a plane. As I say to my friends, "I'm comfortable in my own shoes and in my own skin. I don't need stilettos to turn heads. However, if they're on sale, and make me look thinner, then I'll consider them."

This brings me to our next secret weapon at menopause. With the sense that life is not a dress rehearsal, many women in menopause start to live the mantras, "Good is good enough" and "Stop sweating the small stuff," especially when it comes to their appearance. Are we more practical and pragmatic? Absolutely. We know how to choose our bat-tles. We know how much effort we're willing to expend. We know by now what works and what doesn't. Which way is best? I have friends and patients whose menopausal beauty routine consists of a little dab of Oil of Olay morning and night and a regular haircut. I also know plenty of women who have their plastic surgeon on speed dial with fewer wrinkles than a newborn baby. Ah, that's the beauty (pun intended) of this issue. It's your own personal choice. Is there one way to approach how we view our outward appearance at menopause and beyond? Of course not! Each of us must find the path that feels right and suits our life and lifestyle.

Meet three women—Corinne, Deb, and Michele—whose changing skin and concerns about appearance represent a range of what many of us are coping with as we transition through menopause—from wrinkles and acne to worrying about dark spots and moles. You may recognize yourself or a friend in these stories.

CORINNE'S STORY

Corinne's northern European ancestry combined with her love of sun wor-shipping during her teen years left her with dark brown fallout from sun damage. Brown blotches pebbled her face, neck, and hands. Though she managed to mask most with a concealer, every morning she sighed as she faced her reflection. Her skin tone was uneven and what used to be cute freckles were now similar to the dark liver spots her grandmother and mother had. She scoured the drugstore for products that promised to lighten her skin and spent a fortune on pots and potions, creams and lotions. The trouble was, she couldn't remember to use them regularly and was always running out of the house before she remembered to put on more sunscreen. She felt out of place wearing a hat except at the beach. She'd use the creams for weeks, and then she'd be crestfallen when just twenty minutes out in the light of day without sunscreen would erase weeks of diligence.

Corinne felt like it was a losing proposition and that she should just give in and give up. She was also concerned that some of her dark spots could be more worrisome moles and be early signs of skin cancer. During her annual exam, I noticed a few questionable areas on her back, and because she had a family history of skin cancer, I referred her to a dermatologist. I knew that Corinne would need "mole mapping."

With mole mapping, a series of approximately thirty-five to forty digital photos of the entire body are taken. In this way, individual moles can be magnified and examined and compared to photos from previous "maps" taken of the body. I knew that with the number of moles Corinne had, that she'd most likely need to have these types of photos taken every six months.

While visiting the dermatologist, Corinne asked about the options to help her lighten her skin and get a smoother, clearer complexion. She left the dermatologist's office with samples to try at home and brochures outlining various procedures to help eliminate brown patches and uneven skin tones. Corinne settled on using prescription-strength creams for several months to lighten her brown discolorations. Her mole mapping revealed a few suspicious areas that luckily were completely benign and not cancerous. Her sunscreen use improved and within six months, she saw a moderate but noticeable improvement. She also learned some quick makeup tips, which she could apply in less than three minutes. All of it helped restore her glow and her confidence.

DEB'S STORY

Deb came to see me for her annual exam just as her periods were beginning to become more irregular. She had a few hot flashes and night sweats, but that wasn't what she was most concerned about. In the last few months, her skin had completely forgotten that she was forty-nine, not seventeen, reverting back to high school with acne and breakouts. Her own personal oil production had ramped up, producing pimples, especially around the time of her periods.

Deb remembered dealing with her problematic skin during her pregnancies, too. "There's a lot on my back. I can barely see it and I can't reach it," she said. "How am I going to get the acne cream between my shoulder blades?" Deb was embarrassed about her skin. "My back is all pebbly and red, and I'm self-conscious undressing in front of my own husband. What's happening?" she asked.

Deb borrowed her teenage son's acne washes and drying agents, which helped a little, but it was still distressing to have her otherwise smooth complexion time-travel back to adolescence. She knew that teenagers often went on the birth control pill to treat their acne, and she was happily surprised when I suggested that because she was a nonsmoker and had normal blood pressure that she was also a good candidate for a low-dose pill. The pill had another benefit—helping with her irregular periods. Within three months, her acne had receded and her periods became more predictable.

MICHELE'S STORY

Michele had the kind of infectious laugh that everyone loved. She not only appreciated a good belly laugh but also knew how to tell a bawdy joke. No one expected the petite woman with an angelic face to have a ribald sense of humor, which made it more fun. She was hilarious, and she knew it. There was only one downside that she could think of: the laugh lines and crow's feet that were the marks of a life of laughter and fun.

Since menopause, she noticed with a frown that her laugh lines were deeper and her crow's feet were permanent. "Damn," she thought. Her sunny personality didn't suffer too much from worrying about a few wrinkles, but still, she was a little sad that her face had more creases. Michele loved the way her mother and grandmother had aged. Their faces told a story of lives full of love and laughter. She wanted that, too, but the wrinkles made her look a lot older than she felt.

Michele was a high-school math teacher. Facing her teenage students every day, she envied their smooth, wrinkle-free, fresh faces, but she didn't envy the myriad challenges that lay before them. Each day at school, she looked out on a sea of young faces and never once thought about trading places. Michele knew about treatments that made wrinkles magically disappear but also knew that they were expensive. "I'd rather go on vacation," she reasoned. Though a few of her friends had dabbled with Botox, fillers, and plastic surgery, it wasn't the path she wanted to pursue. Still, when she came for her annual visit, she wanted to talk about her crow's *feet. After reviewing the available options, she decided that injections and procedures just weren't her style but wanted to keep the information tucked into her purse, just in case she changed her mind.*

THE NITTY-GRITTY ON YOUR SKIN

Although prevention is the key to having a healthy glowing skin, by the time you're in the throes of menopause, any sun damage that occurred ten to thirty years ago is probably now exhibiting itself with dark spots, patches, and discolorations. Compounding the problem, estrogen, which may be fluctuating wildly during the perimenopausal transition, stimulates the skin's pigment-producing melanocytes. These cells respond by increasing their production of darker pigment. It's interesting and distressing that you can get an overall tan from sun exposure, and yet also have scattered areas with much darker spots or areas that seem to have shifted into overdrive with brown discolorations. As time goes on, the combination of years of sun exposure, hormones, and your own body's genetic predisposition all conspire to cause annoying discolorations.

Hormonal fluctuations are also responsible for an increase in acne and hair growth at menopause. Never doubt the power of hormones! As estrogen levels swing from one extreme to another, our androgens, or male type hormones, such as DHEA (dehydroepiandrosterone) and testosterone, can also fluctuate. These androgenic hormones influence how the hair follicles respond, causing unwanted hair growth as well as increased oil production and acne.

The passage of time also brings a loss of collagen in the skin, leading to deeper lines and less elasticity. As the skin loses its natural pliability and ability to spring back, momentary wrinkles that come from laughing, frowning, or other facial expressions become permanent reminders. The lines may be few or many. They may be thin and barely visible or deep grooves that leave a permanent impression.

Natural Solutions for Looking Your Best

Before, during, and after menopause, looking your best can take a lot more time and effort. Want to guess what the best available beauty treatment is that helps restore a healthy, vital appearance? Hands down, the absolute best beauty treatment happens to also be the one that's been proven in countless studies to decrease the risk of cancer, diabetes, heart disease, and other serious medical conditions. It's something that's available to everyone, everywhere. What is this miracle treatment that's been around for centuries that restores a healthy, sexy appearance and a healthier body? Still not sure? During menopause and the years after, the best way to improve your appearance is to . . . wait for it . . . surprise: Get regular exercise! Really!

Exercise, which can be as simple as walking around the block or as involved as training for a triathlon, is the best beauty treatment available. Not only does it help you keep your weight down, exercise also releases feel-good chemicals known as endorphins, leading to a healthy glow, more confidence, enhanced sexiness, and less risk of serious health issues. During menopause, making the time to get your blood pumping, increasing your heart rate, and working up a sweat with regular exercise is the first and best option for improving your appearance. A healthy glow is sexy!

Sexiness is all about attitude and confidence. Tweaking our appearances so that we like what we see boosts our confidence. The beauty is that every woman will have her own ideas about what she's willing to do to look and feel her best. What follows are a few options and strategies for some of the challenges that often show up during menopause.

Hydrate and Moisturize

No matter what your beauty regimen is, staying well hydrated with plenty of fluids is one of the easiest ways for your skin and hair to look great. Soft, smooth skin comes from applying lots of moisturizer regularly. Moisturizers don't add moisture to the skin, instead they create a barrier that helps retain moisture and prevent drying and flaking. It really doesn't matter what you use—drugstore brands or high-priced designer creams from specialty stores. The most important thing to remember is to use whatever you like, but use it regularly to keep your skin soft and smooth.

Sleep

Getting seven, eight, or more hours of sleep each night will strengthen your immune system and help your skin cells rejuvenate naturally. There's no substitute for looking healthy and refreshed than getting regular sleep. When you're sleep deprived from being up all night with night sweats, your skin will look haggard and the dark circles will be more intense. Getting more rest through long stretches at night or power naps during the day helps you feel and look your best. Resting is just as important if you can't sleep.

Nurturing Yourself

In our culture, there's so much emphasis on outward appearances that many people overlook the beautiful glow that can only come from the rich inner work and personal growth that nurtures who we are. Menopause is often the first time in a woman's life that she gives herself permission to take care of her own needs and make herself a priority. As you nurture yourself by making time for the pursuits that you enjoy, your happiness quotient will increase, which plays out in your confidence and how you appear on the outside.

Diet

Everyone knows that you are what you eat, and that's because it's true. Beautiful, healthy skin and hair starts from the inside. When we eat five to seven servings of vegetables and fruits each day, the vitamins and nutrients contribute to overall health, and it really shows up in our skin and hair. It's better to spend more time and money on a healthy diet before looking into expensive creams. You'll look and feel better from eating salads and lots of colorful vegetables than from applying the latest cream or serum at night.

Improving the Skin You're in with Traditional Treatments

Acne, dark patches, wrinkles, and sagging skin are common complaints for menopausal women. There are treatments available for each of these issues—from creams, peels, and injections to plastic surgery and liposuction. All can help you look and feel your best.

When it comes to acne, the list of available treatments is virtually endless. Many creams and prescription products use tretinoins, also known as retinoids. These vitamin A derivatives work by helping the cells exfoliate and turn over much faster, which decreases the production of oils. They also help by preventing skin cells from accumulating oil and forming blackheads.

Women who are headed toward menopause and are still having periods are considered perimenopausal. For those women who don't smoke, have normal blood pressure, and are healthy, birth control pills are an option that helps smooth out the wild swings in hormonal fluctuations and helps decrease oil production, thus improving acne. At all ages, any acne treatment can take a few months to see an improvement.

Where dark patches are concerned, there are also many treatments available to lighten darker areas and restore a smoother appearance. Options range from creams, lotions, chemical peels, and light and laser treatments to dermabrasion. All of the treatments for discolorations work to interrupt the function of melanocytes and decrease the production of darker pigment in the skin. None of these treatments can restore the skin to the smoothness and perfection of a newborn baby's without any risk of complications or trade-offs. These treatments are good, no doubt about it, and they absolutely improve appearance; however, there are the risks of rare but possible side effects to consider, such as skin reddening, loss of elasticity, and scarring. It's also important to have a realistic expectation of how much improvement you'll see.

Treatments for wrinkles and sagging skin are designed to help restore the smooth appearance of the skin. Some treatments work by counteracting the loss of collagen that occurs naturally as we age, and others stop muscles from creating fine lines. Many treatments speed up skin rejuvenation, which can partially restore a younger appearance.

Let's take a look at the various treatments available for skin issues common in menopause.

Creams for Dark Patches

There seems to be an infinite number of creams and topical agents that lighten the skin and help remove discolorations by interfering with the action of the melanocytes. Lower doses are available without a prescription at most local pharmacies, from direct sales online, or directly from the manufacturers. The most potent and effective are only available with a prescription. Many prescription products use several ingredients in combination. Some incorporate retinoids (derivatives of vitamin A) and hydro-quinone, which are used for many different skin conditions, including acne, rosacea, and improving dark patches.

Improvement with these treatments may take between four to eight weeks. Though results vary, most women will see a 20 to 70 percent improvement. Common complaints about using creams are sensitivity to the ingredients, the length of time needed before improvement is seen, and the need to use them daily.

Chemical Peels for Dark Patches and Acne Scarring

These treatments work by removing the top layer of skin and stimulating new, less pigmented cells to replace what was "washed away" by the peels. Chemical peels rely upon relatively weak acids that decrease the amount of pigment in the cells. Two of the most common acids used are glycolic acid and alpha hydroxy acid.

Often, a skin-lightening cream with hydroquinone will be recommended before and after the chemical peel to enhance its absorption and effectiveness. Because some darker-skinned women may see a worsening in their condition after a treatment, it's important to do a patch test first on a smaller area of skin. The most common side effects are redness, infection, and irritation of the skin. Some women may also develop cold sores after treatment.

Phototherapy for Dark Patches, Rosacea, Wrinkles, and Acne Scarring

Phototherapy uses light to heat the cells just below the skin's surface, causing these cells to regenerate and replace surface skin cells much faster than normal. Phototherapy also helps skin cells produce more collagen, which reduces wrinkles and eliminates dark patches and some of the tiny blood vessels near the skin's surface that lead to redness and rosacea.

- **LASERS**—The word "laser" actually stands for light amplification by stimulated emission of radiation. In this case, the word "radiation" refers to high-intensity energy that barely enters the skin and is absorbed where the cells produce color (chromophores). The absorption of energy from the laser destroys the chromophores. The depth that a laser penetrates is controlled by the wavelength of the light emitted. Lasers are effective at eradicating dark pigmented areas. Some of the most common side effects include pain at the time of treatment, redness, irritation, mild swelling, and cold sores.

As with a chemical peel, some women will exhibit more pronounced pigmentation in the skin after treatment, so it's important to have a patch test first on a smaller area of skin before undergoing extensive laser treatment.

- **INTENSE PULSED LIGHT (IPL)**—This recent development takes laser treatment one step further. Instead of continuous intensive light therapy delivered to the skin, pulses are used to decrease the total exposure. The pulsed light barely enters the skin and is absorbed where the cells produce color (chromophores). The absorption of energy from the pulsed light destroys the chromophores. The depth that this intense pulsed light penetrates is controlled by the wavelength emitted. Intensive pulsed light is effective at eradicating dark pigmented areas. Some of the most common side effects include pain at the time of treatment, redness, irritation, mild swelling, and cold sores.

  As with a chemical peel, some women will exhibit more pronounced pigmentation after treatment, so it's important to have a patch test first on a smaller area of skin before undergoing IPL treatment.

- **FRACTIONAL PHOTOTHERMOLYSIS**—Fractional photothermolysis, also known as Fraxel, takes laser phototherapy to yet another dimension. Fraxel works by using both heat and light (laser) to treat the areas of dark pigmentation. Instead of using all laser to affect the pigment-producing cells, Fraxel only emits a fraction of the typical amount of laser energy compared to what's emitted with traditional laser treatment (approximately 15 to 20 percent). The rest of the energy emitted is in the form of heat, which causes less damage to the surrounding normal skin. It's thought that, in this way, healing occurs faster and there's less risk of side effects. Some of the most common side effects include pain at the time of treatment, redness, irritation, mild swelling, and cold sores..

  As with any of the treatments, some women will exhibit more pronounced pigmentation in the skin after treatment, so it's important to have a patch test first on a smaller area of skin before undergoing Fraxel.

Dermabrasion and Microdermabrasion for Dark Patches, Acne Scarring, and Wrinkles

Both of these procedures help the skin exfoliate and rejuvenate faster. Dermabrasion uses a fine sandpaper, laser, or carbon dioxide to remove or abrade away the top layer or layers of skin to help smooth away fine, small wrinkles, acne and acne scars, discolorations, even tattoos. Dermabrasion is considered a surgical procedure and is typically completed in one session with the help of a local anesthetic. The skin rejuvenates in weeks or months and, in the meantime, is quite red and raw looking. People look as if they have a severe sunburn as the skin heals. Side effects include dryness, irritation, pain, itching, and sensitivity to the sun. Some women may also develop cold sores.

Microdermabrasion differs from dermabrasion in that it doesn't remove as many layers of skin and is much gentler with fewer possible side effects. With microdermabrasion, there's often a scrub with fine gritty particles that's applied to the skin first, and then what looks like a minivacuum cleaner sucks up the exfoliated skin cells. Sometimes the microdermabrasion machine also applies a soothing serum or cream after the exfoliation. Microdermabrasion typically requires several sessions to notice improvement and is not as effective in reducing the appearance of discolorations.

Botox for Wrinkles

Botox is a purified form of the botulism toxin and works by paralyzing muscles. Botox is given in miniscule quantities directly into the tiny muscles of the face that produce crinkling around the eyes, frown lines between the eyebrows, worry lines on the forehead, and thin lines around the lips. It takes two to three days to temporarily paralyze the muscles that were injected and wears off within three to six months. Because everyone's facial musculature is different, some people will have a paralysis that causes an unintended lift or droop in other muscles. If that occurs, the effects are temporary and will resolve in a few months.

Fillers for Wrinkles

The most popular types of fillers are composed of hyaluronic acid, which is injected in very small quantities directly into the creases and lines of the face. Fillers immediately help plump the area and smooth away lines without paralyzing the muscles. They partially or completely "fill in" the deep grooves that seem to drag the mouth and face down. Fillers can be mixed with a local anesthetic to decrease the pain with injection. Fillers can last six to twelve months. There are also permanent fillers that have more potential side effects, such as clumping below the skin and permanent changes in appearance.

If you're considering using fillers, do talk to a board-certified dermatologist or plastic surgeon to help you choose the one that's best for you.

Plastic Surgery for Wrinkles and Sagging Skin

There are many different kinds of procedures that are available, and new techniques are being perfected all the time. These surgeries are evolving as women and men search for a more natural look and less obvious corrections. There's a range of different options available. Mini facelifts only tighten a few muscles or segments of the small muscles in the face. With mini facelifts, the results are much less dramatic and contribute to an overall impression that the person is much more well rested and looks good for their age without looking as if they've obviously had work done.

Liposuction for Sagging Skin

With age, the neck area can start to resemble the waggling wattle of a turkey's neck, or fill in with fat pads. Aging can produce jowls and sagging from the jaw to the neck. Liposuction of the chin and neck can create a smoother appearance and help define the contours. Many plastic surgeons also suggest a neck lift to tighten the muscles in the neck, which prevents the appearance of noticeable bands or cords that extend from the edge of the chin to the middle of the neck producing a ridge-like appearance.

There are also many different procedures that are available to completely reconstruct noses, cheeks, or chins. Lips can be plumped, foreheads smoothed, breasts augmented, and everything else you can imagine.

Besides neck and facelifts, there are eye lifts, brow lifts, breast lifts, butt lifts, and you name it. If you were born with or acquired something you're not thrilled with, then it most likely can be improved upon. If you decide to proceed, then by all means get a second and even third opinion.

Nurse Barb's Secret Beauty Tips

Free and Instant Facelift Prescription

STEP 1   Smile.

STEP 2   Tilt your chin down slightly.

STEP 3   When you smile touch the tip of your tongue to the roof of your mouth. This pulls your cheek and chin muscles up and reduces the appearance of wrinkles.

STEP 4   Keep smiling and repeat as necessary.

Preventing Discoloration

- Use sunscreen and sunblock at 30 SPF or higher, even on cloudy days.
- Stand in the shade.
- Wear a hat.
- Bring along a light-colored umbrella when you know you will be outdoors.
- Wear sunglasses.

Lightening Dark Patches

These are the most effective ingredients in preparations used to lighten skin:

- Hydroquinone
- Kojic acid
- Mandelic acid
- Retinoids: tretinoin and adapalene
- Azealic acid
- Niacinamide
- Soy (in topical creams)

For Injections

- **TO FIND THE BEST CLINICIAN**—Ask friends who've had these procedures so that you can see their results.

- **USE AN ICE PACK**—Apply it to any areas you plan to have injected to help numb the pain and decrease discomfort.

- **ASK FOR A NUMBING CREAM**—Emla (a numbing cream) can be applied to the area that will be injected one-half hour before the injections to decrease discomfort.

- **TRICK YOUR BRAIN**—Concentrate on squeezing your hands or applying firm pressure to another area of your body, like pressing into your thighs or palms to confuse your brain's perception of the pain.

To Prevent Cold Sores After Procedures

If you're planning to have a chemical peel, laser, Fraxel, intense pulsed light, or dermabrasion, do the following:

- Be sure to ask the clinician for a prescription of Valtrex, an antiviral medication to take for three to seven days. Here's why: when the skin is irritated, it's more likely to respond with an outbreak of oral cold sores.

- Even if you've never had a cold sore previously, you may have the virus that causes cold sores lying dormant in your body. These treatments may reactivate the long-dormant virus, which can lead to an outbreak of cold sores. The antiviral medication is a safe way to prevent painful and large cold sores from marring your appearance.

DISCOVERING INNER BEAUTY

"Beauty is more than skin deep." This quote is especially apropos for women around menopause. You now have the secret weapons at your side. You have the confidence to walk in your own inner beauty and stride with pride into your own future. Confidence is a powerful aphrodisiac, increasing the appearance of vitality as well as upping the sexiness quotient. You've also got a healthier and more realistic perspective. You know that things are changing and there's only so much you can do, but you have the wisdom and experience to know how to work your assets and highlight your best features.

And finally, you're practical. You don't have time to sweat the small stuff. Good is good enough, and there's so much more out there that you want to experience. You'll look great, because you feel great. It also takes inner work to make peace with our bodies and with our reflections, which despite our wishes to the contrary are changing. I admire women who are comfortable with themselves, rolling with the wrinkles, graying hair, and changing shape. I also admire women who decide that they'll look the way they like, thank you very much, and will do whatever is necessary so that their outward appearance more closely resembles their inner vision.

3

Facing the Hairy Truth About Menopause

$\mathcal{A}$t menopause many women begin to notice some not-so-subtle changes in their hair. There's too much hair where they don't want it and not enough where they do. It's distressing, confusing, and maddening. The texture and color are also likely to be different as hormonal changes play out in our hair. Many lucky women have great hair throughout their lives: terrific texture with never a wayward hair on chins or necks. It's pure luck, and picking the right grandparents, of course, because genetics plays a huge role. Then there's the rest of us, who might see a shadow on our upper lips or coarse dark hairs sprouting from our chins. We may notice that our hair is thinner on our heads and that there's more left swirling in the shower drain or in the hairbrush.

When it comes to our hair, we all ask girlfriends for advice on which salon to go to, which products will help, and how they deal with challenges. Meet Emmi, Ann, and Shelley, who had very typical issues with their hair during menopause.

EMMI'S STORY

Emmi had beautiful thick, dark, arching eyebrows and long dark lashes. Each morning, she had her tweezers at the ready, searching in the magni-

fying mirror for any stray hairs that had sprouted up overnight, threatening to mar the perfection of her brows. Each month, while getting her hair colored at her cousin's hair salon, she had her face and eyebrows waxed and threaded. Being of Iranian descent, she was no stranger to the best ways to remove unwanted hair.

Since menopause, her chin was driving her mad. As she drove to work each day, she'd stroke her chin, feeling for any telltale stubble. It was embarrassing, because, without the magnifying mirror, she could barely see it, but knew that anyone under forty could. She remembered being distracted when she visited her grandmother and not being able to listen because she was focused on the long, curling chin hairs that grew from her grandmother's neck.

Emmi knew it was crazy, irrational, and vain, but she often fretted about who would take care of her hair removal when she was an old lady in the rocking chair. She shuddered at the thought of having stubble and any long, coarse, curling hairs like her grandmother. At times, she felt like the bearded lady at the circus. In addition to regular waxing and threading, she was considering electrolysis and laser hair removal but was having trouble justifying the high cost.

When Emmi came in for her annual exam, she asked about treatments for unwanted hair. I laughed because I'm of Italian descent, meaning that I, too, am no stranger to extensive and regular hair removal. For many women of Mediterranean and Middle Eastern descent, the thick gorgeous eyebrows are a package deal and come with an unwanted predisposition toward finding dark, coarse hair around the chin and neck that gets worse at menopause. There are other hidden surprises, too, including lots of hair where we don't want it. Moustaches, sideburns, hair on our chins and neck! Hello, magnifying mirror. When in doubt, be sure to have your tweezers at the ready.

When I looked at Emmi's chin and neck, I could only see a few dozen hairs scattered around the entire area. Unlike some of my other patients, who have hundreds of hairs and would be good candidates for laser hair removal, I could see that Emmi would have good results with electrolysis, which was much less expensive. She found that within three months of regular electrolysis visits, she was completely free of dark stubble and only used her tweezers for her eyebrows.

ANN'S STORY

Ann was also battling extra hair on her chin during menopause, and because of her African American ancestry, there was an added challenge. Ann's hair tended toward a more natural curl, which meant that as it grew out of her chin and neck, it tended to curl in on itself, becoming ingrown and creating a small pimple. As these pimples burst, they left dark patches and slight scarring. Ann hadn't noticed this prior to menopause, but then, as her hormones fluctuated, new facial hair started to sprout up. She resorted to tweezing and shaving. "It's hard to feel sexy when you have stubble," she explained.

I recommended a step-by-step approach for Ann that began with using warm soaks to soften her skin and help the ingrown hairs find a natural way out. In addition, opening up her pores also allowed some of the natural oils to be released. Next, I recommended that she try a prescription cream, Vaniqa, that works directly on the hair follicle to slow down the rate of hair growth. Because her hair was dark and coarse, she was also a good candidate for laser hair removal, which is even more effective when used with Vaniqa. Within six months of using both treatments, her chin hair and ingrown hairs were markedly reduced, and she felt much more confident and sexy with her partner.

SHELLY'S STORY

A successful author, Shelly was constantly in the public eye. Her book tours took her all over the country, and she made frequent appearances on local television. To her great distress, despite having access to hair stylists and the best hair-care products, Shelly was losing her hair. At first, she noticed that the individual strands of hair weren't as thick, and seemed softer and finer. As her other menopausal symptoms became more noticeable, her thinning hair also became more apparent. There was so much daylight between strands that eventually her scalp became more visible as less and less hair grew. Shelly knew that most of the women in her family had very thin hair and most had developed hairstyles to masquerade their hair loss. Shelly had been tested for physical causes for her hair loss, including low vitamin D and low thyroid hormone levels, but the verdict was disappointing—there was no physical reason that could be reversed. Instead, she had female-pattern hair loss—androgenetic alopecia.

Shelly was devastated as her scalp became more visible. She tried increasing her vitamin intake and learned how to comb hair from the sides of her head over the top. When she came to see me, she wanted to talk about solutions. It was some consolation to know that over 3 million women also suffer from female-pattern hair loss, and that it's probably not related to menopause but happens coincidently in the fifties and sixties. After reviewing her lab tests, we talked about increasing her vitamin D intake and using Rogaine (minoxidil) at the prescription strength.

Shelly used Rogaine for several months and noticed some improvement. She didn't expect to have a thick head of hair overnight but was still happy to find that her scalp became less and less visible as more hair grew in. She wasn't completely satisfied, and so we discussed another idea that had worked for many of my breast cancer patients who had lost their hair due to chemotherapy. As you might have guessed, I suggested that she buy a good-quality wig.

Initially, Shelly was shocked, but after talking it over with friends, visiting a wig boutique and trying on a few styles, she made the decision to get one. Initially, she only thought of having her wig as a backup for special events, but after wearing it a few times and hearing all the compliments, her confidence soared and she began to wear it more and more. At home and with friends, the wig gave her an option as the Rogaine worked its magic to help her hair grow back. Shelly's hair did eventually grow thicker, and many of her bald spots filled in partially with fine, soft hair. Her hair wasn't completely restored, but at least now she had more hair to work with. And Shelly now has several options. She can go natural or choose different wigs depending upon how she wants her hair to look that day.

THE NITTY-GRITTY ON HAIR

The hair we see on the outside of the skin is only a tiny portion of the entire length of the individual hair. There's approximately one-sixteenth to an eighth of an inch of hair that lies just below the surface of the skin embedded in the hair follicle. The hair follicle holds what appears to be a tiny bulb of hair at the very end. When hair is removed by plucking, waxing, or threading, it normally takes six weeks to three months for the hair follicle to completely reactivate and produce a new hair. Even though you'll see new hairs cropping up every day, each follicle needs time to rest, recharge, and replace the strand of hair.

Hormonal fluctuations are responsible for an increase in hair growth on the face, neck, and chin at menopause. Never doubt the power of hormones! As estrogen levels swing from one extreme to another, androgenic, or male-type hormones, such as DHEA and testosterone, can also fluctuate. These androgenic hormones stimulate more rapid reactivation of hair follicles that may have been asleep prior to menopause. As the androgenic hormone levels fluctuate, women may notice a sudden crop of a few dozen new chin hairs. Women who notice a sudden change or extreme amounts of new hair growth should see their healthcare practitioners for evaluation as this may signal a more serious hormonal fluctuation from an overactive ovary, thyroid gland, or adrenal gland that's not a result of menopause. Women who notice more hair growth may also notice that their skin is oilier and their adolescent acne has returned. Thankfully, most of these beauty challenges can be managed with a few tips you'll find in this chapter.

It's not clear if these androgenic hormones also play a role in female-pattern hair loss, which is likely an inherited condition. Although hair loss is more common in the fifties and sixties and may be related to aging and not hormonal changes, many women start to see evidence of hair loss in and around the menopausal transition. Hair loss can become much worse if there's an underlying thyroid disorder, celiac disease, gluten intolerance, or vitamin D or vitamin B deficiencies.

Before any treatments are initiated for hair loss, it's important to evaluate and screen for those conditions first. I've had many patients see a vast improvement in the thickness and amount of hair on their head when their underlying thyroid and celiac disorders were discovered and treated. I've also seen countless patients with low vitamin D levels, less than 32 ng/ml, who've been happy to see a marked improvement in the quality and quantity of their hair once their vitamin D levels reach 40 ng/ml or higher. Likewise, it's important to look at any chemicals, dyes, straightening agents, or other hair-care treatments that may be leading to more hair loss. Diet and smoking also play a role in hair loss. A healthy head of hair depends on good overall health and nutrition.

. . . .

Nurse Barb's Great Hair Tips

- If you're losing your hair around menopause, ask your healthcare provider to do the following blood tests, which could indicate an underlying condition: TSH (thyroid-stimulating hormone), free T4 (thyroid hormone level), thyroid antibodies, celiac panel, vitamin D levels, and vitamins B6 and B12 levels.

- If you're already on thyroid replacement, ask your healthcare provider about also starting T-3.

- If any vitamin values are low, start a supplement. At the very least, start taking a multivitamin.

- Consider using Rogaine (minoxidil), which may take three months before any noticeable improvement occurs.

- Reduce the styling products and heat you use on your hair.

- Find a good stylist who can help you find a style that's flattering.

- Wigs look more natural now than ever before, so experiment with a new wig or two.

. . . .

Nurse Barb's Hair-Removal Tips

- Prevention is the best strategy for unwanted hair removal. Before the hair turns gray, consider laser treatment, which only works on dark hair. Unfortunately, gray hair doesn't have any pigment and thus can't absorb the heat from a laser, which means that the gray hair will continue to grow even if the area is treated with a laser.

- Electrolysis is another effective permanent solution; however, some hair follicles need to be zapped several times. Use Emla anesthetic cream prior to electrolysis to reduce the pain.

- Vaniqa is a prescription product that helps slow down hair growth. It also works well when combined with laser treatment.

- Threading and waxing are effective ways of pulling out hair by the root. However, this can cause the hair to grow in thicker and coarser over time.

- Contrary to what you've heard, occasional shaving when you can't wax or use other better methods won't cause permanent, thick, coarse stubble. Regular shaving, however, isn't a good long-term solution due to the upkeep.

- Invest in a good magnifying mirror. As you become more dependent upon reading glasses, you won't be able to see offending hairs as easily in a regular mirror.

• • • • • • • • • • • • • • • • • • •

YOUR CROWNING GLORY

You can go anywhere with great hair. Healthy hair is sexy, and yet, we only want hair where we want it. We crave lots of thick luxurious hair on our heads but are loathe to see even one on our upper lip or chin. During menopause and beyond, women with smooth, hairless faces may be surprised to see a few stray hairs pop up from nowhere. These are easily remedied with a pair of tweezers. If there are more than a few hairs, then other more effective measures might be needed.

There are many things that can influence how your hair feels and looks. If there are any underlying health conditions such as a thyroid disorder, celiac disease, or vitamin deficiencies, the evidence will be apparent in the hair. Healthy hair depends upon a healthy diet and avoiding the overuse of hair products and heat. But never fear; as you've learned, there are many options that really work to decrease and eliminate unwanted hair as well as remedies for sparse and thinning hair.

4

Satisfying Sex and Avoiding the Status Quo

*S*ex is a hot topic all the time, but even more so during menopause, with the roller coaster of hormones, physical changes, and
relationship issues all colliding at the same time. Add to that the fact
that a women's sexual response cycle is more complicated than a NASA
space mission and you get a recipe for complexity that can boggle the
mind.

No matter where I go, as soon as women learn that I work in women's
health, they invariably ask me about sex. No matter where I am, whether
it's on a plane, a train, at a wedding, a funeral, or a dinner party, friends
and perfect strangers alike take the opportunity to ask the questions that
they can't ask anyone else. As soon as someone finds out that I work as
a nurse practitioner in women's health, it's almost as if a big red "Will Talk
About Sex" sign blinks on my forehead. It's no longer shocking because
everyone has questions about sex.

Underneath the millions of questions about sex that I've answered
over the years, there's one underlying question that everyone, yes, *everyone,* has. It's especially true in menopause, when everything is changing.
Everyone wants to know, "Am I normal?"

Let me answer you right here, right now: Yes, you are. No matter if you
are having sex three times a day or once every three years, you are normal. Yes, you are normal as long as—and here's the big caveat—you're

comfortable with your experience. If you're happily celibate and haven't thought about sex in months, you're normal. If you're in a relationship and want to have sex more than your partner, you're normal. If you're self-sexual, whether in a relationship or not, and using masturbation and/or a vibrator as a release every day, you're normal. If you're interested in sex one to two times a year, you're normal. If you're hot for your partner every day, you're normal. If you're just interested in cuddling, you're normal. If you like to read trashy romances and fantasize about George Clooney (and really, who doesn't like to think about George Clooney?), then, you guessed it, you're normal. If you like men, women, or both, or like being by yourself—yes, you're normal, and what's more, you're in good company.

I hope I haven't left anyone out, and if I did, then let me just say this, you're normal, too. If you've probably reached the conclusion that pretty much anything and everything is normal, you're right, because it is.

As women, we are wonderfully complex. We are not machines with on/off switches that trigger sexual desire and satisfaction. Thank goodness! Our bodies, hearts, and minds are interwoven and interconnected, especially when it comes to sex. Our unique blend of hormones is different from men's, which means that our senses respond differently to images, scents, touch, words, tone, inflection, actions, and our own thoughts, just to name a few. We can become aroused simply by reading an erotic section of a bodice-ripping novel or from seeing our partner empty the dishwasher without being asked. We can be turned off by unresolved anger or by the thought that our teenagers are in the next room. During menopause, it can take longer to have an orgasm. Orgasms may be a pleasant yet slight tremor, or they can be rocking and rolling earthquakes of passion. By the way, both experiences are, you guessed it, normal.

In my exam rooms I hear many women's stories about challenges with sex. Here are just a few normal women with normal challenges that I'd like to share with you. I hope Vanessa, Wendy, and Tracy's stories will help you feel that you're not the only one who is dealing with a new or unexpected situation in the bedroom.

VANESSA'S STORY

Vanessa had always enjoyed having sex several times a week. Since she began noticing the occasional hot flashes one to two times a week, and some irregularity in her periods, she also noticed a big increase in her sex drive. "I always liked to have sex," she confided. "But I'm driving my husband crazy. He can't keep up with me. Look, it's great, but what is going on here?"

Vanessa also complained of more breast tenderness and more clear, vaginal discharge. She found it odd, though, that despite the feeling of being wet all the time, she often needed to use a lubricant because her vagina seemed a little dry. Vanessa was happy and yet also a little perplexed. It didn't take much to ignite feelings of arousal, from seeing an Abercrombie and Fitch billboard to stealing a peak at some of the more muscled guys at the gym lifting weights. Her husband was game and a good sport at first, but after a few months, he was tired and searching the Costco vitamin aisle for zinc supplements to replenish what he was losing from all the fun time in the sack.

Vanessa found that she seemed to want sex a lot during certain times in her cycle, when she thought she might be ovulating. When her periods were irregular, her sex drive went into overdrive. "I seem to always be ready and willing and that's a big difference for me." Vanessa was happily surprised that her sex drive ramped up so much so fast.

"It's really not a problem," she confided. "I just want to know if this is normal and if I need to be worried about anything." Since she was still having her periods, Vanessa could still become pregnant; however, with her husband's vasectomy, she didn't need birth control. I reassured her that she was indeed quite normal. We discussed why she had this sudden increase in sex, and I gave her some samples of lubricants to try. "I know that even though I'm ready and willing every night, my husband is tired. Instead of initiating sex at night, when he's likely to ask for a rain check, I set my alarm so that we can have sex in the mornings," she said. "That way we both start our day with a smile."

WENDY'S STORY

Wendy hadn't had a period for at least a year, although it might have been a bit longer. She couldn't remember exactly; she was just glad that they were gone. Though many of her friends had hot flashes and night sweats, she was one of the lucky few who seemed to sail through menopause with few symptoms. A bubbly and friendly woman, Wendy worked full time as an accountant in a large firm and had been happily married to Drew, her second husband, for over nine years. Her kids were in college, and she was always thinking about her next vacation. At the moment, she was learning French so that she could take a cooking course in Paris that focused on chocolate.

She loved chocolate, although you'd never guess from her waistline, which she kept trim by exercising at the gym and taking her dog for twice daily walks. She had so much more time now that her kids were launched. Wendy loved her life, her family, and her job, but there was just one issue nagging at her, and it was too embarrassing to bring up.

When she came in for her annual physical exam, she didn't indicate that there were any questions or concerns. Unlike dinner parties or other occasions, where people always ask about sex, when it comes to physical exams, less than one in five people bring up the topic of sex with their healthcare providers. Amazing but true! Understanding that fact, I know that it's my responsibility to bring up this very personal and private concern in a way that communicates that it's safe to talk about sex, and I won't judge what I hear.

Wendy told me that her interest in sex had disappeared virtually overnight. "One minute it was there and then the next, poof." She waved her hand. "It was gone, just like that. The trouble is, I don't even care. Sex drive, what sex drive?" she asked rhetorically.

Wendy loved her husband, and they were very affectionate with each other. If he initiated sex, she felt ambivalent. On one hand, she knew it was important to stay connected, but on the other, she'd just as soon go to sleep. I suspected that Wendy was perfectly normal because diminished libido and sex drive is a common concern in menopause. I asked her to do a few lab tests for anemia and thyroid hormone levels to rule out any underlying cause. During her exam, I used a mirror to show her how her vagina had changed. The elasticity and normal pink folds had virtually disappeared and the skin was much drier. I asked her to consider using a small amount of vaginal estrogen to help restore the elasticity and lubrication (see Chapter 8).

We then talked about some specific suggestions to regain some intimacy with her husband. Wendy decided to start by using a tried and true, very simple strategy: she would "Make a Date for Sex." Although this sounds simplistic and obvious, it works. Women are surprised because though they put everything else on their lists, sex is one activity that most of us assume has to be spontaneous. Making a date for sex and putting it on the calendar can put the spark back into any relationship.

After she started using estrogen treatment in her vagina, she noticed an increase in her natural lubrication and more thoughts about sex. Wendy was game to try scheduling sex, and soon she found that instead of having a take-it-or-leave-it attitude, she was acting more like she did ten years earlier. The combination of vaginal estrogen and scheduling sex helped ignite some dormant sexy thoughts and fantasies she'd forgotten about.

Wendy told me that just by acknowledging that sex was on the table, so to speak, she began anticipating and fantasizing more as the time approached. It was like looking at a menu of mouthwatering descriptions of food, where the anticipation heightens the enjoyment of the experience. Knowing that she'd be lighting a few candles and wearing something sexy also helped her get in the mood. Once she and Drew got the engine started, she revved up and found that her desire also increased. Although it took a bit longer to have an orgasm, they were still very satisfying sexual experiences.

As an added bonus, Wendy liked how much more emotionally connected she felt to her husband, which led to more spontaneous encounters in addition to their scheduled dates. She felt less and less that sleeping was preferable to connecting with her partner sexually and that taking the extra time to get the party started was well worth it. Wendy confided later that she had even shed the practical, everyday, granny panties that she used to wear, trading them for hotter and sexier versions. Just putting on silk and lace underwear helped remind her of the fun in store for later that evening.

TRACY'S STORY

Tracy worked long hours and traveled so much that she didn't have time for a relationship. She knew that she was married to her work, but that didn't mean that she wasn't interested in love. The trouble was she was never in one place long enough to start more than a superficial relationship. She wasn't interested in quickie encounters, and she knew herself too well to think that she'd ever be comfortable talking about the possibility of sexually transmitted infections in a casual relationship.

There were plenty of temptations on the road and even more opportunities, but Tracy didn't just want sex; she was interested in finding a loving relationship. It would have to be the whole package because she wasn't ready to give up the idea of romance. A few years back, she tried online dating and met lots of men, but the trouble was she couldn't quite sync up her schedule with theirs and most of the good ones had moved on. Tracy wasn't at all interested in letting the lack of a partner interfere with her being self-sexual. Even though she was always a little worried that TSA would search her carry-on bag and discover her vibrator, she never left home without it.

Tracy was using an estrogen patch to control her hot flashes and night sweats, and she noticed that her vagina and the labia around it were getting a bit drier. Unlike in the past, when she could have an orgasm in just a few minutes with masturbation, now that she was menopausal it seemed to take forever, until a friend suggested that she try a vibrator. In the past, before discovering the joys of battery-operated sex, there were times that she just threw in the towel and gave up. "Whoever invented vibrators should get a medal," she laughed.

She was also disappointed that her orgasms just didn't have the same intensity or power as they did in the past. As she reflected back, Tracy knew that a lot had changed. She wasn't ready to completely give up and wave good-bye to a healthy and satisfying sex life, and she wanted to know what she could do. Like Wendy, Tracy was beginning to show the signs of vaginal dryness (see Chapter 8). She decided to add some vaginal estrogen to her routine and began by using a cream twice weekly. Within a month, she had much less dryness and was delighted to find that her orgasms were a lot more powerful and intense.

THE NITTY-GRITTY ON SEX

Our sex drive is influenced by a number of physical, emotional, and hormonal factors. Estrogen is the main hormone that influences libido or sex drive in women. During perimenopause, there may be wide swings in estrogen levels, which can cause a roller coaster of varied levels of sexual interest. During this hormonal transition, the range of sexual interest is amazing—from little to no interest to an obsession with sex. It depends upon many factors but especially upon the levels of hormones that are bathing the woman's brain.

Other androgenic hormones also play a role in influencing libido and sexual response, including testosterone and DHEA, which are secreted by both the ovaries and the adrenal glands. They're known as androgenic hormones because they are present in much larger quantities in men. When the brain is bathing in estrogen and androgenic hormones, women are more likely to be interested in sex, have more fantasies and sexual thoughts, and be more receptive to potential partners.

Although many women would welcome an increase in libido, some women may be uncomfortable with a sudden surge in sexual interest and may wonder if what they're experiencing is normal. Menopause can bring so many unexpected physical and emotional changes that an increase or decrease in sex drive is perfectly normal, natural, and expected. If you're one of the lucky women like Vanessa with plenty of sexual desire and power surges of libido and lusty thoughts, my best advice is to enjoy this gift and have a good time.

On the other hand, I know many women who are thrilled and surprised by a sudden surge in sexual interest around perimenopause and menopause. It can be an unexpected bonus but may also complicate and add undue pressure in a relationship with a partner who may or may not be able to keep up.

However, as menopause progresses, estrogen levels will decline if a woman is not using any hormonal treatments. As estrogen and other hormone levels spiral down, it's quite normal to experience an abrupt loss of sex drive and libido. It's almost as if our libido decides to take a prolonged vacation and forgets to send a postcard. This may be a welcome relief or cause distress. Many women like Wendy are surprised because they had plenty of sexual thoughts and fantasies prior to menopause and didn't expect to see those thoughts diminish without so much as a wave good-bye. But don't get discouraged, and don't give up if you want things to change. There are practical and proven options in menopause to help regain a healthy and vital sex life. Sex can be a complicated dance between partners. It's not only okay to ask for help if you're feeling over-whelmed, but you have nothing to lose and everything to gain by talking to your healthcare provider or a licensed sex therapist about any issues that seem too difficult to overcome on your own.

The Brain-Body Connection

Our brains are our most important sexual organ, and without a constant stream of libidinous hormones like estrogen, progesterone, and testos-terone, the brain can become indifferent to sexual stimuli. For women at midlife, this often means that they're not as receptive to sexual signals that lead to arousal and a willingness to consider sex. Sexual desire and being receptive to the idea of sex are a complicated series of dance steps, where any number of factors can interfere with a woman getting in the mood and then continuing toward sexual fulfillment.

As if there weren't enough going on, our brains and bodies are so inti-mately connected that nearly anything can derail a woman's desire for sex and her ability to enjoy sex once she does become interested and aroused. It's too noisy or too quiet, she's angry or overworked, the phone rings or the dog barks—you name it, *anything* can interfere.

Unfortunately, as long as the list of interfering factors is, any change in hormone levels can prevent the journey from even starting. Becoming aware of some of the barriers to a satisfying sex life in menopause is the first step in removing them and finding more satisfaction.

When it comes to how the genitals react to hormonal changes, the story becomes more complicated. As a woman journeys through menopause, the estrogen receptors in the vagina, vulva, and clitoris all play their part. As estrogen levels decline, these receptors become more and more thirsty for estrogen. As the supply of estrogen diminishes and becomes scarce, the receptors in the genitals become more discouraged and dormant, eventually giving up on replenishment. Without estrogen to nourish them, these tissues also start to change. The skin becomes more dry, less able to lubricate and stretch, and less able to respond to touch, images, or thoughts. Before menopause, when the genitals are literally bathed in estrogen and other hormones, just seeing an image of something hot and sexy could initiate lubrication, but as estrogen levels decline, the ability to "get wet" also declines.

The good news is there are many ways to help regain satisfying sexual health. Number one on the list is to follow the old cliché "Use it or lose it." Whether a woman uses hormone treatments or doesn't, it's critical for vaginal health to remember to pay attention to your genitals regularly, with intercourse, manual stimulation, oral sex, masturbation, or vibrators. Sexual activity increases blood flow to the area, which in turn helps keep you and your vagina healthy and happy.

There are many women who have frequent sexual experiences well into their seventies and eighties who never use a lubricant and who don't require any medication or treatment.

Natural Ways to Get the Party Started

Increasing blood flow to the genitals will help rev up your vagina for satisfying sex. Some ways to increase blood flow include soaking in a hot tub, taking a hot bath, applying warm packs to the area, and using warming gels. There are many different arousal gels available that contain niacin as the active ingredient. This B vitamin dilates the blood vessels when applied to the genitals. Niacin increases blood flow, which in turn helps get the party started by improving both arousal and orgasms. The most common side effect is a burning sensation.

Increasing Vaginal Moisture

One of the most confusing topics regarding vaginal health is what exactly the difference is between a vaginal remoisturizer and a vaginal lubricant. Lubrication is what the vagina produces during sexual arousal to further increase the amount of moisture and to help anything that's inserted glide in without discomfort. Vaginal remoisturizers are used daily to help the vagina *make* its own lubrication; however, they are not lubricants. For any woman of any age, keeping the vagina moist all the time prevents the skin from feeling dry and irritated.

For menopausal women who don't want to use hormones, there are a number of vaginal remoisturizers available over the counter (see Chapter 8). The more moist the vagina is, the more likely that its pH levels will stay low (more acidic), meaning less irritation and less chance of an infection. Vaginal remoisturizers are also one of the only options available for women being treated for breast cancer who are undergoing chemotherapy and can't use estrogen. Some chemotherapeutic medications, such as aromatase inhibitors, make vaginal and vulvar dryness much worse.

Increasing Vaginal Lubrication

A decrease in vaginal lubrication is often the first sign that menopause is approaching. Many women are bothered by vaginal dryness and the feeling that their vaginas are smaller, tighter, and less flexible. Though there may be some lubrication, it's often far less than what a woman previously experienced. There are an almost infinite variety of vaginal lubricants that can be used with partners or with toys. See my tips at the end of this chapter for my recommendations.

· ·

Make a Date for Sex

Put sex on your to-do list. Add it to your calendar and set aside the time for sex. Whether you're with a partner or you're self-sexual, anticipation can get the arousal cycle in gear. Because a woman's sexual response cycle is complicated and influenced by many external conditions, anticipating sex can help shift a woman's gears from being sexually neutral to sexually receptive. It's much more difficult to go from 0 to 60 mph without filling up the gas tank first. Women are deliciously complicated, our brains respond to a variety of signals, and simply reminding yourself that you're going to have sex can help your body get ready. Putting on special clothes, reading erotica, lighting a few candles, massaging lotion onto your skin, or watching a movie can all set the stage and help you develop a hotter, sexier mood.

· ·

Prescription Options for Improving Dryness and Pain

Many women want to avoid using prescription treatments to treat dryness and pain with sex; they prefer to use more natural remedies. But this condition never improves on its own; in fact, it gets worse. That's why I often recommend that women consider the benefits of prescription treatments because the risks are low.

Vaginal Estrogen

With more estrogen receptors in the vagina and vulva than anywhere else in the body, even a small decline of estrogen in and around menopause will have a negative effect on the vagina and also on sexual response and orgasms. This condition isn't temporary and doesn't improve with time or after menopause passes. Unfortunately, vaginal dryness gets worse if left untreated. The full benefit of estrogen treatment takes a few weeks, though most women will feel better in a few days. The process that caused the dryness occurred over months and years, so though it would be nice if we could wave the magic wand and presto, have a moist, pink, receptive vagina overnight, the reality is that it takes six weeks for the estrogen receptors to fully wake up and another six weeks to feel the maximal improvement in lubrication and sexual response.

Vaginal estrogen is available as a cream, as a small tablet (Vagifem) that's inserted into the vagina, or via a vaginal ring that slowly releases estrogen over three months. The most common side effects are breast tenderness and headache.

• •

Understanding Risks: Vaginal Estrogen Versus Hormone Treatments

One reassuring aspect to the use of vaginal estrogen preparations is the amount of estrogen is significantly less than what is used with hormone treatments for hot flashes and night sweats, meaning the risks are also much less. In fact, there is so much less estrogen in vaginal preparations that there's no need to also take additional progesterone to prevent overgrowth of the uterine lining, bleeding, and abnormal cell growth. In addition, research has not shown any increased risk of breast cancer, stroke, heart disease, or any other serious health risk with the small amount of estrogen that's recommended for use in the vagina.

Vaginal estrogen is used for several different circumstances to help maintain the health of vaginal tissue when estrogen levels decline. For example, many new moms who are breast-feeding find that their vaginas are dry, more prone to infection, and uncomfortable. This occurs because the hormone (prolactin) that stimulates milk production in breast-feeding inhibits estrogen. Women who are past menopause also benefit from a little added estrogen to the vagina.

Though there are no studies that have looked at whether vaginal estrogen increases the risk of breast cancer recurrence, many women with a history of breast cancer have opted to use it after discussing their options with their oncologist. The risks are theoretical, while the benefits are known. Some women decide not to take any risk, and others decide to use vaginal estrogen to improve the quality of their life. Each woman in this situation should talk to her oncologist and her gyn practitioner about the risks and benefits so that she can make her own individual choice.

· ·

Ospemifene

A new medication, ospemifene (brand name Osphena), an oral tablet taken once daily, was recently approved by the FDA for women who have vaginal dryness and painful sex. Ospemifene is a selective estrogen receptor modulator (SERM), which is unique in that it has positive estrogen effects on the vagina specifically, improving vaginal health and moisture, while having antiestrogen effects on the breast. It's important to know that like vaginal estrogen, this medication has not been studied in women with breast cancer, so any woman with a history of breast cancer must discuss the risks and benefits of taking ospemifene with their oncologist. The most common side effects are hot flashes and vaginal discharge.

Vaginal DHEA Suppositories

Vaginal DHEA (dehydroepiandrosterone) suppositories are being studied currently in ongoing clinical trials. DHEA is a hormone produced by the adrenal glands and is also sold as a supplement in health food stores and pharmacies. Some healthcare providers recommend DHEA for women with vaginal dryness who can't use estrogen. It is believed that DHEA is converted into estrogen within the vaginal tissues. Though not approved by the Food and Drug Administration (FDA) yet, promising research from Europe shows that women with a history of breast cancer who used vaginal DHEA suppositories had significant improvement in their symptoms of vaginal dryness and did not experience any significant side effects.

Testosterone

Testosterone is another of the important hormones that influence sex drive. A woman's adrenal glands and ovaries produce testosterone before menopause. After menopause, testosterone and other androgenic hormone levels decline as ovarian production ceases and leaves the adrenal glands with the task. It seems logical to try to replace the lost testosterone, which would theoretically increase sex drive.

In Australia and some European countries there are approved testosterone formulations available for women; however, that's not the case in the United States. While women wait for a safe testosterone treatment that's on the approval list from the Food and Drug Administration (FDA), many are resorting to using compounded testosterone or testosterone medications that have been approved for use only by men. Using testosterone is not without its potential side effects, which can include a deeper voice, increased hair, clitoral enlargement, more irritability, and changes in cholesterol values.

• •

Nurse Barb's Recommended Lubricants for Hot Sex

- **OLIVE OIL/ALMOND OIL**—If you can eat it, cook with it, or drink it, you can use it for smoother sex.

- **CARRAGEENAN**—This is a water-based lubricant derived from seaweed and helps increase smooth sliding with intercourse, while also reducing friction. You can find it on MiddlesexMD.com.

- **LUVENA**—This is a unique formulation that's very slippery with cranberry extract and no preservatives, which helps maintain the delicate pH of the vagina.

- **LIQUID SILK**—This is a water-based lubricant with a little silicone mixed in, which provides the best of both types of lubricant. It has a silky feel that lasts a bit longer than straight water-based lubricants.

- **ASTROGLIDE**—This silicone-based lubricant was developed by NASA but not for sex in space—although it can help take you and your partner to new galaxies of fun!

- **OH! WARMING LUBRICANT AND K-Y WARMING GELS/LIQUID**—These products contain niacin, which helps increase arousal.

- -

Nurse Barb's Tips for Smooth Sex

- **IF YOU'RE HAVING PERIODS**—Be sure to use contraception as pregnancy is still possible.

- **HAVE AN ORGASM FIRST**—If there's pain with entry and things feel a little too tight, try having an orgasm first to help the vagina stretch and elongate.

- **OPEN WIDE**—If you bear down, like you're having a particularly difficult bowel movement, your vagina will open up and widen. This makes it easier to insert fingers, toys, and partners.

- **GET THE JUICES FLOWING**—Increase blood flow to your genitals by taking hot baths, using a shower spray directly on genitals, or using a hot pack or heating pad set on low.

- **GET WET**—For vaginal dryness, make your genitals more slippery with lots of lubricant.

- **DON'T TEAR**—Lubricants help to avoid tearing and stretching your delicate skin, which would dampen even the most enthusiastic woman's desire.

- **SAMPLE SLIPPERY LUBRICANTS**—Try different kinds of lubricants to find the one that works best for you. Keep a small washcloth or towel nearby so that you can have fun without worrying about staining clothing or sheets.

- **WHEN IN DOUBT, CHECK IT OUT**—If you're experiencing any vaginal itching, burning, unusual discharge, or any urinary symptoms, do see your healthcare provider and hold off on intercourse, which can make a bad situation a lot worse.

- **THERE'S LOTS TO GAIN AND NOTHING TO LOSE IF YOU ASK FOR HELP**—For other sexual issues that are more complicated, consider seeing a licensed sex therapist.

- **ORDER ONLINE**—There are lots of great resources, including one developed just for women at midlife: MiddlesexMD.com. Many women feel more comfortable shopping for lubricants, toys, and other intimate products from the privacy of their own home.

• • • • • • • • • • • • • • • • • • • •

FROM GOOD TO GREAT SEX

Good and satisfying sex is a wonderful part of life. Though there may be a few challenges during menopause, none are insurmountable if the desire is there. Women who use hormones and those who don't can still have deeply satisfying sexual experiences and intimate relationships. No matter what your sexual experience in menopause, it's normal to wonder if you're normal. I can assure you that you are, in fact, normal. If you do have challenges, don't be discouraged; as you've learned, there are a few easy adaptations that can help you regain your interest and your enjoyment, which is well worth the effort.

5

Taking the Two-Way Street of Intimacy

*I*f you're not having the kind of satisfying sex you crave, you're not alone. There are multiple forces conspiring against us, especially at menopause. Everyone wants the kind of wild, hot, romantic, playful, creative sex we read about in novels or see on the big screen, and yet it seems elusive and out of reach for us mere mortals. Virtually every midlife woman I speak with fantasizes about out-of-this-world, fantastically fun sexual experiences, and yet when she wakes up back on earth, in her day-to-day existence, she would be happy with just a little undivided attention and an emotional connection. Sex that was more satisfying would be icing on the cake.

Satisfying sex is not out of reach no matter if you're in a relationship or by yourself. Many women are very self-sexual through vibrators and/or masturbation. This is perfectly normal and natural. If you're wondering if you're the only one, don't. Just about 99.9 percent of all of us are self-sexual. And in case you're wondering, I have it on good authority that even some nuns are self-sexual. Surprised? Don't be. It's normal. So let go of any guilt and consider yourself in good company.

If you're in a relationship, perhaps you're one of the few lucky ones, having lots of mutually satisfying, hot, creative, and fun sex with a partner, or you may be like millions of women who wonder if they're the only ones *not* having sex. At midlife, just as we're hitting our stride, feeling more confident and powerful than ever before, when we're appreciative of peak experiences, the reality is that many of us aren't having peak experiences in the bedroom and feel frustrated and unfulfilled with our drab sex lives. Thousands of women have nagging doubts about themselves and their partners. They wonder if there's something wrong with their energy levels, their interest, their anatomy, or the way they respond. They are shocked to wake up one day with barely a fantasy or thought about sex. Yet it doesn't take much for most women to get turned on, and millions yearn for a more satisfying sex life. A more satisfying sex life is within every woman's reach, whether she has a partner or is by herself. This chapter will cover some relationship issues that many women at midlife encounter.

Let me invite you to a virtual "girls' night out" where you'll meet three women who have a lot to say about relationships, sex, and intimacy during menopause. Tanya, Carmen, and Mindy are all navigating issues that are common at this time of life, and each has found their own path to a more satisfying sex life.

TANYA'S STORY

Tanya made a nice dent in her first martini and smiled as she listened to her girlfriends trade stories. The topic was—what else? Sex. A friend who was recently single was explaining the minefield of relationships with much younger men whose heartbreakingly smooth and beautiful bodies were so perfectly intimidating that it was impossible to undress in front of them unless the lighting was confined to one small tea light candle. "It's hard to relax and have fun when you're worried about whether they've noticed the cellulite and stretch marks," she said. Another friend chimed in with her take on sex with men at the opposite end of the age spectrum. Older men had their own flaws, from tons of emotional baggage and landscapes of wrinkles to health issues and hopeful little prescription bottles of Viagra. Where were all the men that weren't too old or too young, but like Goldilocks's search, just the right age and stage for fun time without having to rely on two margaritas just to work up the courage to take off your clothes?

As the stories continued, Tanya was fascinated. She'd been married for over twenty-five years, and her husband was still nudging her in the middle of the night a few times a month. She tried to explain to him that nudging wasn't foreplay, thank you very much. His response was to bring flowers home regularly. It was very sweet and endearing but didn't quite measure up to what she really wanted. If only he'd be a little less clueless and take a few minutes to listen to her talk about her life and her day, or acknowledge all the little things she did to make his life easier. Maybe she'd be more in the mood if instead of assuming that she was utterly captivated and enthralled by his recitation of the trials and tribulations of his work, he took the time to listen to her.

She was unfailingly polite, but underneath her smile she was seething with resentment. She felt that since she automatically sensed when he needed to talk through something, that by now, he should be able to figure out that she also needed the same consideration. He was clueless when it came to checking in with her. She also resented having to constantly remind/nag him, feeling that by now, he should be able to figure out that the dishes didn't wash themselves and his stack of clothes didn't magically get put away.

Tanya was completely comfortable with her husband. She didn't have to worry about what he thought of her body or that they'd both put on a few extra pounds. They had sex about once a month, usually after Tanya had a glass of wine to relax. She just wished she could shake him into being more considerate of her needs. Why couldn't he be more like her girlfriends, who knew how she felt, or would notice when she just needed to talk?

When Tanya came in for her annual, she and I talked about the age-old question that women have been grappling with for centuries, "Why can't men be more like women?"

We talked about how difficult this situation is. It's both unfair and unrealistic to expect our partners to be able to read our minds and anticipate our needs. As women, we have a different set of communication skills than our partners. Just because we can anticipate what our partners are thinking and feeling doesn't mean that they have the same ability with us.

Women often feel resentment building because they assume two things. One, that their partners know what they need, and two, that they're purposely withholding it. It's number two that leads to heaps of resentment. Once we work on those assumptions, most women are genuinely and happily surprised that with a few simple communication techniques, their relationships improve. I recommended that Tanya practice "I messages" that foster communication and avoid the accusatory "You messages" that impede real dialogue. I gave her an "I message" example from my own marriage and shared an exchange between me and my husband:

"I feel frustrated when we can't agree on what to do over the weekend. I like to plan ahead, but I know you prefer to be more spontaneous. It would helpful if you could give me some idea of what you'd like to do so that I can get a better idea of what I can get done."

After our conversation, Tanya told me that she tried communicating more specifically with her husband. For her, the perfect setup for sex would be having her husband listen intently to her talk about her day and ask questions about how she felt without trying to solve or fix the issues she just needed to vent about. To her credit, she had approached him with this request, which was met with, "I thought that's what girlfriends are for."

That started a little heated back and forth, but she was proud of herself for responding, "Hey, I listen to you drone on and on about the most inane issues you have at work. You could return the favor, just listen, and then you might get lucky a little more often. Get a clue!" She went on, "It's really simple! All you have to say is 'Really? And then what happened?' And then you actually have to listen, or pretend that you care about what I'm saying. That's it! Just listen to me!"

It didn't happen overnight, and she had to remind him to give her equal time, but within a few months, they'd established a new pattern. As Tanya felt more heard, she felt a stronger emotional connection. It wasn't long before she was nudging her husband, which was a happy surprise for both of them.

CARMEN'S STORY

Carmen's clenched smile barely hid her disappointment as she listened to the same old story through her phone. While she was running to get to work on time, her partner was busy rehashing yet another botched job interview. Carmen was doing everything she could to hold it together and not explode. She was trying to be encouraging, but the evidence was piling up. It was her worst fear come true—her partner, Ella, was never going to get a job.

She wouldn't even apply at the local coffee shop that offered decent benefits, saying that it wouldn't look good on her resume for the more managerial work she was qualified for. At this point Carmen didn't care what she did. Ella hadn't worked in over five years. Carmen would be happy if Ella could do something, anything, that provided their family with a few extra dollars and lessened the stress she felt from shouldering all the burdens of supporting everyone. When she wasn't working, Carmen was paying bills or worried about paying the bills.

Carmen was so angry that Ella was the last person she wanted to have sex with.

"I know that I'm part of the problem," Carmen confided. "And that I'm enabling her by picking up all the slack." Carmen not only worked full time but also did most of the cooking and shopping. As she described how things had changed when Ella had been laid off, I ventured that Ella might be depressed and should see her primary care provider for an evaluation. "I've begged her," she said. "She won't see anyone. It doesn't matter what I say or how much I plead. I'm done. In fact, I've started sleeping in the guestroom."

Carmen took my advice and started regular counseling with a licensed therapist. No matter what she ultimately decided to do, she'd need support in communicating with her partner, if for no other reason than to make it easier to be the kinds of parents that their children needed. No matter if she decided to stay or go, she'd need emotional support and help with more effective communication strategies. After a year of counseling, Carmen realized that their issues extended past the bedroom and she decided to leave Ella.

Carmen started dating about eighteen months later. "The big difference between the old me and the new me," she related, "is that I feel like I can ask for what I need, and I'm more aware of the importance of sharing everything."

MINDY'S STORY

Mindy and her husband slept in the same bed but hadn't touched each other in over two years. She wanted to have hot sex the way they used to when they first met, but he wasn't interested. She would have gladly settled for snuggling in his arms, but that was also off limits. They were good parents and talked about all the things that went along with having a house and kids in school, older parents, mortgages, work, paying bills, and what to do on the weekends. On the surface, they probably seemed like a happy, well-adjusted couple, never arguing in public. She felt that, everywhere but the bedroom, they were a happy compatible couple. The reality was they were more like roommates than lovers. She knew that he loved her, but there was one big thing missing. There was no physical affection. None, nada, not even a hug in the morning. Any attempt she made to touch him, hold his hand, or even reach out for him was rebuffed. He had never been cold and distant in the past. After reading self-help books and taking the ubiquitous surveys in women's magazines, Mindy thought she had a working diagnosis. She was pretty certain that it all stemmed from one small issue that had grown into the elephant in the room and was the one thing he refused to discuss. The last time they tried to have sex was over two years ago, and he hadn't been able to get an erection.

For the first few months, she had tried to reassure him and he'd been receptive to trying oral and manual stimulation, but when that didn't work, he became more discouraged and withdrawn. He gave up. He didn't want to discuss it with her, and the more she suggested that he see his doctor, the more stubborn and angry he became. After a while he started rebuffing any attempts she made toward hugging or cuddling. It was almost as if any touching reminded him that it didn't lead to the sexual promised land, so he nipped it in the bud before it got started. Any time she even approached the subject she was met with stony silence, so she gave up. Now she understood the saying, "Two ships that pass in the night." He was a cold fish that she was ready to wrap up in newspaper and leave behind. Masturbation a few times a week, while not exactly what she wanted, was better than nothing and it was a good release.

Mindy didn't think that they needed counseling, because they didn't fight and she didn't think he was cheating on her. But despite being married, she was very lonely. They weren't connecting sexually or physically at all. It was sad, and she wondered if this was how it would be for the rest of their lives.

"It's so depressing," Mindy told me. "I don't want to give up sex. I'm only fifty-four." Her sex drive was alive and well. She wanted to have sex, though she was tired of being rejected by her husband. She felt like her marriage had turned into a case of "The Right Kids and Wrong Husband."

Mindy and I talked about safe ways that she could bring up the subject of their sex life. I gave her some simple scripts she could use to gently discuss the "elephant in the room," which sounded like erectile dysfunction.

Later, she told me how she went to his man cave and closed the door so that the kids wouldn't hear them. "Look, I know this is difficult for you," she began. "But it's difficult for me, too. I don't want to live like this anymore. I love you, and I want to be more connected emotionally and physically. We don't have to give up on sex and having fun in bed. It's not too late. You don't seem happy, and I know I'm not happy. I'm willing to try if you are. It's not okay with me for us to continue to live like roommates."

Mindy told me that, after her husband's initial resistance, he agreed to see a sex therapist. Within weeks of seeing the therapist, they had made a lot of progress with emotional and physical intimacy. The first thing the therapist had them do was work on their communication, which helped as they worked on the physical aspects of their sex life. Mindy thought that their communication was fine prior to seeing the therapist, but soon realized that there were big gaps that needed to be filled before they could connect in the bedroom. After a lot of encouragement from the therapist and from their improved communication, her husband finally agreed to talk to his primary-care physician about medications for erectile dysfunction.

Although it's a very slow process, my experience is that these deep and complicated issues take lots of time and baby steps. The way people interact with each other doesn't change overnight. It does take time and is well worth the effort.

THE NITTY-GRITTY ON SEXUAL RELATIONSHIPS

Don't believe sex surveys. One of the reasons so many people feel inadequate about how often they're having sex is the regular reporting of results of surveys on sexual frequency. Every few months, we hear from well-intentioned researchers that the frequency of sex is holding steady at three times a week. No matter what a person's age or the length of their relationship, time and time again, we hear that people are having sex three times each and every week.

The biggest problem with sex surveys is that people lie! Yes, they lie! Really. People lie when asked how often they're having sex. If you've read a sex survey that says that couples over forty are having sex three times a week, don't believe it. Seriously, don't believe it! People *think* that they *should* be having sex three times a week, so that's what they mark down on sex surveys. No one wants to feel ashamed or inadequate, even in an anonymous survey. I've seen results from ninety-five-year-olds who are in a rehab facility, who still check off the box that says three times each week. For the record, I do have a few patients in their nineties who are having regular sex, but they are the happy exception, not the rule.

To get to an accurate reflection of sexual frequency, researchers found that they needed to ask the question a little differently. If they ask, "When was the last time you had sex?" then they get a better and more accurate idea of the real frequency of sex. Ready for the answer? The average sexual frequency for couples who have been together for more than one year is once every three weeks. No kidding.

The only people having sex three times a week are teenagers and college students, but of course, not your teenagers or college students! If you have a mortgage, at least one of you works outside the home, and you've been married for more than two years, *and* you're still having sex once a week or more often, then guess what? You're LUCKY. In fact, you're incredibly lucky that you're getting lucky so often. But please, don't gloat, because a lot of your friends are in the midst of some serious dry spells.

Let me just congratulate you and your partner, because it takes a lot of work and a lot of luck to stay that connected for the long term. Consider celebrating by having even more sex. For the rest of us, let's talk a bit more about frequency.

Let's Talk Frequency

People often ask me what's the normal frequency of sex in a relationship. The way I answer is with another question, "How often would you like to have sex?" It's the word "normal" that makes this question impossible to answer. And that's because there is no one standard or normal frequency of sex. Frequency of sex is dependent upon an infinite number of factors, from a person's age to their general physical and psychological health. The reassuring and short answer is that there is no normal frequency of sex to use as a guide and measure our own sex lives against.

We have a skewed and inaccurate perception about how often we *should* be having sex. Notice that I used the word *should*. That's because in our society, we place too much emphasis on standards, benchmarks, goals, and what's perceived as normal. No one wants to be abnormal, so we strive to meet the suggested frequency, and if it doesn't work out that way, few people are willing to admit it.

We're constantly bombarded with images and messages about sex. Every sitcom couple is having sex or talking about having sex in each episode, and every detective show and drama weaves sex into the plot. Women's magazines have sex surveys, sex columns, and sexual how-to articles. We see people on TV talking about sex constantly, and it's no wonder many of us feel inadequate. Everywhere we look, it seems that everyone else is having lots more sex than we are. What's wrong with us? Why can't we be going at it like rabbits? Why are we too tired? Why are we more interested in a good night's sleep? Where is that elusive sex drive that we took for granted in our teens, twenties, and thirties?

Instead of focusing on how often people are having sex, what I like to focus on is whether or not a woman is bothered by what's happening or not happening in her sex life. If she's happy and fulfilled having sex twice a year—on her birthday and anniversary—and that's what works for her, then there's no need to intervene, admonish, or suggest that she should be doing anything differently. (We'll talk about what to do when a partner wants to have sex more frequently a little later in this chapter.) On the other hand, if a woman is frustrated and unfulfilled in her sexuality and wants things to change, then there's lots that can be done to help her reignite her sexual spark and have a much hotter, sexier menopause.

What Is Average at Midlife?

The average frequency of sex for couples at midlife is about once every three weeks, which works out to about ten to fifteen times a year. That's not to say that you should be having sex every three weeks—it's only an average. I'm not saying that it's normal or a frequency that couples, regardless of circumstances, should aim for. It's just the average when you consider the range of people having frequent and infrequent sex.

As you'd expect, people in new relationships of less than six months have sex more frequently. As the relationship continues, the frequency often decreases. In established relationships of greater than six months, the frequency of sex is likely to be lower when there are stressors from work, family, finances, unresolved relationship issues, health concerns such as high blood pressure or diabetes, caring for elderly relatives, travel, or anything that affects your lives. Let's not forget one of the most important factors: how tired you might be from answering a gazillion emails each day, running a household, paying bills, keeping up with friends, working, exercising, having kids at home, worrying about your kids, worrying about your pets, and everything else. Day-to-day living can be exhausting, leaving little energy for anything but sleep.

If you're not in the lucky group having loads of hot steamy sex, you may take some comfort in these research findings from the *Clinical Handbook of Couple Therapy**:

- Approximately one-third of couples report that one or both has diminished and decreased desire for sex. In fact, this is the most common complaint for couples seeking help with their sex lives.

- 20 percent of married couples have sex less than ten times each year.

- 30 percent of nonmarried couples who have been together for more than two years have sex less than ten times each year.

- Sex therapists define a relationship as a nonsexual relationship if the couples engage in sex less than ten times a year.

Now that you feel better about not being the only one having less sex, don't give up hope for improvement. It's never too late to have more satisfying sex—if that's what you want.

---

*McCarthy B. and Thestrup M. In Gurman, A., ed. *Clinical Handbook of Couple Therapy* (4th edition). New York: Guilford, 2008.

What's a Nonsexual Relationship?

According to sex researchers, if you're not having sex at least ten to twelve times each year, you're in a nonsexual relationship. I think this is a bit harsh and more than a tad judgmental. What if the couple has great sex six times each year? Could they be in a slightly sexual relationship? What if one of them is recovering from an illness, or they're taking care of an elderly relative? Or one is traveling for work? What if they've managed to have great, satisfying, hot sex nine times that year? Is it all for naught, because they didn't have one last quickie? I don't think so. I know from my patients that it's not unusual for couples to have long stretches of time when they're not connecting sexually, and yet because of their deep emotional intimacy, they can pick up where they left off, when the stressors diminish.

You Are Not Alone and You *Are* Normal

I love seeing the looks of relief on my patients' faces when they learn that there are millions of other women out there living happy, busy, complicated lives without sex three times each week. There's nothing to be ashamed about, because when 20 to 30 percent of couples are having sex less than once each month, then we have to redefine normal. What's normal for one couple doesn't work for another.

Many women in midlife find that their interest in sex has disappeared, seemingly overnight. While many are indifferent to this change, many others are bothered and would like to recapture their libido. (This is covered in Chapter 4.)

Being Out of Sync with Your Partner

My patients are also relieved and surprised when they discover that up to three out of every four couples are out of sync when it comes to sexual desire. With those kinds of statistics, you could even say that it's actually abnormal for couples to be in complete agreement about how much sex is just right for their relationship.

Along with the myth of perfect agreement and harmony from each person about the frequency of sex, comes another big myth that gets shattered in midlife. This may not surprise you, but in heterosexual relationships, it's not always the man who wants sex more than the woman. Really! In fact, at midlife, there can be a very jarring realization that the woman's sex drive is far outpacing her man's. As the hormonal roller coaster arrives, many women find that their interest in sex is peaking, just as their partner's testosterone level and libido is starting to decline. Many more women than you'd ever guess are frustrated by their partner's lack of interest.

Hearing "No"

I've heard from many women who find it demoralizing and defeating to be turned down by a partner who's more interested in throwing back a few beers and watching a game than in hitting the sheets together. It takes courage to initiate sex and a strong personality not to feel completely rejected by a "No, thanks." It takes even more courage to suggest sex the next time and the next time after that. No one wants to be turned down repeatedly. Being shut down works on our self-esteem and on how we perceive our shared connection with our partner.

When partners can learn to lovingly decline the opportunity to have sex, while maintaining the emotional connection, both will feel heard, supported, and loved. Neither partner wants to feel pressured, nagged, or guilted into having sex. No one wants to feel manipulated, and yet in a loving relationship, it's reasonable to expect that having sex and talking about sex is an essential part of the relationship.

One script that can soothe some of the hurt feelings might sound something like this, "You know I love you and I'd love to have sex, it's just tonight isn't the best timing. Can we cuddle? How about a rain check for tomorrow or the weekend?" Then it's essential to keep whatever promise has been made. Both partners need to feel loved and respected around this highly charged issue.

Not as Good as It Used to Be

Many women who come to see me also wonder if they should be concerned because even though they are having sex, it's just not as satisfying as it used to be; it is falling quite a bit short of their erotic fantasies about what sex could be. For women, sex isn't just about flipping an on/off switch. Sexual desire, arousal, and intimacy are much more complicated. Women's sexual responses are influenced by a variety of factors, from body image and medical and personal histories to cultural influences and partner concerns.

There are all sorts of other factors that play a role here, too, things like whether it's too noisy or too quiet, do the lights need to be off, is the dog barking, are there kids in the next room who might hear them, are all the bills paid, is the grocery list up to date, and many others. The list of things we worry about is endless, and yet we have to shut all of those other concerns out and focus on our partner and ourselves. It's almost as if all the planets need to be perfectly aligned for a woman to be receptive to sex and be able to relax enough to have an orgasm.

It's not an impossible dream to have a satisfying relationship that's sexually fulfilling. A loving, respectful, and fun-filled sex life is within your reach. It may be easier to achieve than you ever dreamed, but it does take work. Yes, sex can be a purely physical act, and yet for many women, emotional intimacy is a prerequisite.

Secret Sexual Organs

There are a few hidden and secret sexual organs that respond to stimuli, arousal, and thoughts, which many people completely overlook in their quest for more and better sex. So often people focus on the mechanics of sex, how we progress from one phase to the next, that we may forget the secret sexual organs that influence every aspect of the experience.

The most important sexual organs are located much higher on the body than you might suspect. Located just above your neck, your face and your brain are the winning combination that holds the key to sexual pleasure. Thoughts, feelings, and verbal and nonverbal signaling are the manifestations of sexual arousal, interest, receptivity, and enjoyment. When our brains are disconnected from our bodies, the experience is diminished. We can certainly participate in the physical aspects of sex and yet feel frustrated or that there's something missing. If you're wondering how your face fits in here, let me tell you. Your eyes and facial expressions signal to your partner your interest in sex and intimacy as well as whether you're having a satisfying experience or need to make adjustments. Sometimes we feel more comfortable communicating without words, and that's where a wink, a look, or a smile is all part of the sexual dance with our partners.

For women especially, one of the most important aspects of a mutually satisfying sexual relationship is emotional intimacy that comes from respect and trust. In order to be receptive to a sexual experience, many women need to feel an emotional connection first, before being able to relax and allow herself to be aroused and a willing, engaged partner. Without the emotional connection, many women think of sex as ho-hum, take it or leave it, or yeah, whatever. It's the emotional intimacy that can spark the sexual connection *and* be a happy by-product, further bonding us to our partners. The inverse is also true. Without respect and trust that builds an emotional closeness, women are often loathe to connect sexually.

When There's Abuse Present

For women in emotionally, verbally, or physically abusive relationships, mutually satisfying sex is almost never present. It's impossible to trust and allow yourself to be vulnerable if there's any undercurrent of abuse or lack of respect. I've met many women in those situations who start off asking why their sex drive seems to have disappeared when on the surface everything seems fine. As more information about the abuse peeks out from behind curtains of shame, and women talk about how they walk on eggshells just to keep the peace, it's no wonder they are not interested in sex. Abuse tips the scales away from trust, respect, and emotional intimacy—all the necessary ingredients of a mutually satisfying sex life. With an abusive dynamic, most women do need professional help to navigate their way toward a healthier situation.

Anger Kills Intimacy

Unresolved anger and resentment are all too common at midlife with relationships. If there's been an absence of healthy communication where partners don't talk openly and can work out differences, then resentment and anger build. Bickering and sarcasm increase as tensions mount when partners feel less inclined to share and negotiate. Because any communication can lead to a fight, many people either shut down and withdraw or find themselves at each other's throats. If a woman has spent years biting her tongue and not making waves just to keep the peace, by midlife, she's likely to have a volcano's worth of anger and resentment simmering barely below the surface. There may be brief episodes of venting a little, but the real explosion is only a matter of time.

Women in this situation may have expressed themselves and had it fall on deaf ears, or bottled it up. In any case, if a woman is angry, no matter what the cause, it's unlikely that she'll want to have sex and meet her partner's needs. Here's a scenario that many of my patients have described:

"He wants me to be ready for sex when he's ready, which is late at night, after I've worked all day, driven the kids to their practices, gotten dinner on the table, and finally, finally, had a few minutes to myself. Is there ever an acknowledgment or a thank-you? Never. I wouldn't mind, but when I ask him to please pick up a roasted chicken and some milk for dinner, he whines about it and then expects me to thank him over and over because he helped out. Really? I do this every day without one word of acknowledgment, but you help out once in a blue moon and you want a gold medal. Give me a break."

Many women tell me that they feel as if they don't ask for much, and that, when they do ask, it's often met with zero enthusiasm or a grudging willingness, so it's just easier to do it themselves. "I don't want to fight or nag or coax. He should just get off his ass and do it," they complain. I understand this because, like many of my patients, I am also married to an actual flesh-and-blood man and have been for over twenty-five years. I, too, live in the real world where it takes lots of patience, deep breaths, compromise, and the willingness to work on the issues.

COOL AND SEXY SOLUTIONS FOR IMPROVED INTIMACY

Most women are surprised to learn that the key to improving intimacy and sex with our partners doesn't begin in the bedroom. Of course, there are some challenges that are physical or techniques that could be enhanced. However, many more issues arise from poor communication. Improving communication takes work, yet when each partner speaks with respect and feels heard and understood, there's more love, trust, and emotional intimacy, which makes better sex much easier to achieve. Better communication also makes it much easier for couples to lovingly address any physical issues or challenges with technique.

Improving Communication

For many couples, their early sex life might have been focused on what worked physically. However, as we age, there's an inevitable shift in the focus toward more emotional intimacy, which can lead to even greater sexual satisfaction. The most important aspect of sexual satisfaction and physical intimacy begins with emotional intimacy. Emotional intimacy is only possible with open communication and talking about what works and what doesn't—and not just in the bedroom. Many couples find that seeing a marriage and/or sex therapist helps them start communicating about the mundane more easily, which can lead to stronger emotional connections and more satisfying physical intimacy.

Being Specific with Men

It takes two to tango, and it absolutely takes two to communicate effectively in both the verbal and sexual arena. Women and men communicate differently. I know what you're thinking: *Duh!* Yet in the midst of communication that's not working with our partners, we often forget that simple fact. For one thing, we talk more than men do. We use far more words and we work things out by talking. It can be heartbreakingly frustrating or another nail in the relationship coffin to have a partner who, despite many years together, still cannot read your mind or know with a glance what you're thinking. Even if you have the ability to read his mind, he probably can't read yours. Just because you have a nonverbal, emotional shorthand with your friends doesn't mean that your partner can decipher the hidden meanings beneath a raised eyebrow, or what you really mean when you use a different tone when saying the word "really."

How many men anticipate and play through an entire argument in their heads before bringing up a subject? Very few, and yet women do it all the time. Even though you're probably pretty good at reading his mind and can understand what's being said by his raised eyebrow, the vast majority of men are completely clueless and utterly incapable of reading our minds. And if it makes you feel any better, my husband can't read my mind either.

To communicate more effectively and to move past resentment and anger, we need to communicate more specifically with men; otherwise, they have a tendency to tune us out. Most men are eager to please their partners. They just want to know what to do. Here's a common scenario repeated thousands of times every day across our country.

See if this seems familiar to you. A married woman tells her husband, "I need you to help out more around the house." For the woman, she wonders why he's blind to the mountains of chores that are right before his eyes. Why can't he just see all that needs to be done and pitch in without being asked? For the man who hears this request, he's not sure what it means to help out more. It could mean a zillion different things, from setting the table to getting the bills paid, to fixing the leak in the bathroom and everything in between.

Because the request wasn't specific, it's easy for our male partners to become overwhelmed by the sheer volume of possibilities. They don't know where to start, so instead of doing something wrong, they do nothing. If we're not specific, they are unsure if we need them to clean the bathroom or do more laundry. Make lunches for the kids or make dinner? "Help out more" could mean anything.

And there's one more important factor at play here. Without specifics, men also have no idea about your sense of time. Should they get started right this minute or can it wait until after dinner or sometime during the weekend? In order to avoid resentment and seething anger, when asking for something from a partner—be it in the bedroom or in your relationship—it's critically important to be as specific as possible. There's a greater likelihood of your partner understanding and following through if you say something like, "It would be great if you could fold the clothes and put them away by five o'clock, because that's when the neighbors are coming by." You can see other examples of my hot communication tips at the end of the chapter.

Timing Is Everything

A man's sense of time is also different from a woman's. "I'll get to it right away" could mean in the next twenty-four hours or the next two weeks. If you can be flexible with your own timing and choose your battles, the tension will also diminish.

"It would be awesome if you could get to that sometime this weekend," means he has until Monday morning. No one likes a nag, and no one wants to be a nag. However, if there's a pattern of reasonable requests being ignored, then it also helps to be specific. "I don't want to be a nag, and I know you hate me reminding you. It's just hard when I hear you tell me you'll get to it by a certain time and yet it's still not done. What's going on?"

Becoming a Reporter

One communication technique that really helps foster more intimacy is to check your judgmental attitude at the door. Unconditional love means biting your tongue . . . a lot. And sometimes, that means biting your tongue until you can taste blood. Try asking questions as if you're a friendly reporter, who finds the subject fascinating and wants to understand all the factors at play. This requires some emotional detachment from the issue, which is very difficult. However, if you can put your emotions aside and listen without judgment or rolling your eyes or shaking your head or reminding them of their faults and shortcomings, then real honesty and intimacy is possible.

For example, if you are always bickering with your partner about an issue, you might try this approach. This is simplified, but you can insert anything into the examples in quotation marks. "I've noticed that whenever I say the word 'blue' it triggers an argument because you often respond with the word 'red.' I was wondering what happens when you hear the word 'blue'?"

This is a way to open up a dialogue that continues with each partner repeating what they think they heard: for example, "Oh, I see. Whenever I say the word 'blue' it reminds you of a work situation that's annoying, and you're reacting to that, not to me."

The point of the exercise is you can't know what they're thinking unless you find a way to ask that opens up dialogue instead of slamming the door. This takes time and effort and often the help of a counselor, which makes it much easier than doing it on your own.

This is not easy, because every fiber of your being wants to point out how they're wrong, flawed, and hopeless, yet again. It's normal to feel disappointment when our partners are just as human as we are. When we practice understanding and patience, they're more likely to respond the same way.

Addressing Physical Issues

When partners have a physical issue, there's often a psychological component that makes the situation a lot messier. Mindy's situation with a husband with erectile dysfunction is quite common. As our bodies change, so do our partners'. Millions of men over fifty years of age have some degree of erectile dysfunction (ED) that ranges from a complete inability to have an erection to one that only lasts a few seconds. Medical conditions such as obesity, diabetes, high blood pressure, and prostate conditions, as well as the use of medications, drinking alcohol, and stress are just a few of the reasons men at midlife suffer from erectile dysfunction.

There's often a psychological component with ED that may make the situation much more complicated and difficult to treat. As it turns out, when some men have any minor degree of difficulty with sex, they may also have distorted and magnified feelings of inadequacy and shame. These negative feelings and anxiety about performance can become so troubling that their stress about having sex is compounded and magnified even more, becoming a vicious cycle. With the added worry, shame, and feelings of inadequacy, having an erection, which was easy in the past, suddenly becomes an insurmountable hurdle.

Some men with ED are able to have an erection but aren't able to sustain it for more than a few seconds. Even when a partner approaches him in a nonsexual manner, a man may think that it's a prelude to sex, only increasing his feelings of inadequacy and shame. Men in this situation may find any nonsexual touching to be a reminder of what they can't do, leading them to withdraw, avoiding any and all contact.

This type of avoidance leads to hurt and confused feelings that are very difficult to overcome. Although there are a gazillion TV commercials for medications to treat ED, this issue is still shrouded in shame. It takes courage and an acknowledgment of vulnerability to ask for help. If the mechanical issues can be alleviated, counseling can help with the psychological fallout.

$$\bullet \quad \bullet$$

Nurse Barb's Hot Communication Tips

- Avoid making all-or-nothing statements such as: "You never" or "I always."

- Avoid starting any sentence with the word "You."

- Do use "I" messages. These are simple sentences with the following structure:

  "I felt sad/angry/disappointed when I heard you say you weren't going to the picnic. . . ."

  "I was disappointed when I felt that I was being ignored after asking for your help. . . ."

  "I was deeply hurt and worried when you refused to see a doctor about your heart condition. . . ."

- Do follow up the "I" message by asking for what you'd like in a positive way.

"I felt left out and that my opinion didn't matter when you bought that expensive coffeemaker. I'd really appreciate it if you'd call me before you make any more decisions like that."

"I was deeply hurt and worried when you refused to see a doctor about your heart condition. I love you and want you to be around a long time. I'd appreciate it if you'd make an appointment this week."

"I am so sad that we are not connecting with each other emotionally or sexually. I love you and want to work this out. I need for things to be better between us. I'd like to start by making some time just for us each week. Can we start with this Friday night?"

"I feel a little resentful, and like we're not a team, when I feel like I'm doing more than my fair share around here. I know you're busy, too, and I need you to help by . . . "

"Since the hot flashes started, I'm also noticing a lot of other changes, especially with sex. I need a little bit more time to get aroused. It would help if we could use a lot more lubricant and spend more time helping me get in the mood."

- Do validate your partner when he makes an effort.

  "I really appreciate how you got up early to take the kids to practice this morning. You're an amazing father and I love you."

  "It really makes me feel like we're more connected (more like partners) when you listen to me. Thanks."

- For difficult topics, try:

  "It's very difficult for me to be the one in our relationship who has to ask to have sex and who hears 'No thanks.' I'm beginning to wonder if there's more to this and would like to talk more about it."

  "I've noticed that talking about your brother seems to be off-limits in our house, and I'd really like to understand that better. I promise not to make any judgments or say anything negative about your family. I'm just wondering what's going on."

  "It's very difficult for me to be ready for sex at the drop of a hat after working all day and taking care of the kids, paying the bills, and all the

rest. Sometimes I feel frustrated that I seem to be meeting everyone's needs. Do you ever feel like I'm asking too much of you?"

"When I hear the words that you used with the kids tonight, it makes me worry that they're going to tune you out and lose respect for you. I wonder if we could talk about ways that we can both communicate with them more effectively. There's no one right or wrong way here. I'd like to brainstorm some options. Can we do that?"

• • • • • • • • • • • • • • • • • • •

REIGNITING THE FIRE

I know from my own experience and from listening to my patients for over twenty years, that a little respect and a lot of open, honest communication go a long way in fostering emotional and sexual intimacy. Especially at menopause, with all the physical changes that are occurring, feeling loved, cherished, and accepted without judgment is a cornerstone in a happy sexual relationship.

However, if a woman feels that she's the emotional ATM, allowing everyone else to make withdrawals and not having anything left over for herself, it's a recipe for bitterness and resentment. Thorny communication issues don't get better magically or quickly without mutual effort. They didn't develop overnight and may represent deeply ingrained patterns. Have a realistic expectation. This will take time and a willingness to work from both partners. Communication problems aren't easily remedied with one or two conversations. For women who feel as if they're talking to a brick wall, and that their partners aren't meeting them halfway, talking to a therapist or counselor will help you find your voice and the strength to either stay or move on.

I've talked with many women who have made small adjustments in how they communicate with their partners, which have resulted in huge gains. They reap more emotional intimacy, honesty, and deepening trust, which can all lead to the icing on the cake—a much more mutually satisfying sex life. It's in your reach, so give it a try.

6

Understanding the Biology of Menopause

*M*any of my patients are perplexed by what to expect at menopause. Why is their experience so much different from their sisters and friends? Are they normal? Why can't anyone predict what will happen next? Women are understandably frustrated by the lack of consensus and the oft-repeated vague statements they hear such as, "Well, everyone is different," "There's really no way to know what will happen," and "You could sail right through it or have a lot of symptoms."

I understand the frustration and wish there were a "crystal menopause ball" that would enable us to predict what each individual woman will experience. Who wouldn't want to know if they will be one of the lucky ones who barely notices a warm gentle breeze at night, or one of those who has the dreaded hurricane-force hot flashes and night sweats that leave them drenched, exhausted, and irritable?

Just as your journey through your teen years was different from your friends, so is your journey through menopause. I've learned that there's always a story beneath the symptoms and some degree of anxiety behind every question. Most of us just want to know that we're normal and want reassurance that other women not only survived menopause but they also emerged from the other side stronger, wiser, and more confident. I'm here to tell you just that: you will not only survive, but you can thrive now and later.

As you've probably surmised, the most common and bothersome symptoms of menopause are hot flashes and night sweats. Approximately 80 percent of all women will have hot flashes before or around the time of menopause.

Some women have intense, searing heat that builds from their abdomen and travels up to their faces and heads with a racing heartbeat thrown in just to add another layer of anxiety. Others will feel heat ignite at their necks, spread upward toward their scalp, and stand by helplessly as beads of sweat pearl on their foreheads or upper lips.

Hot flashes can manifest as heat radiating out from the chest to the arms. Many of my patients describe feeling as if their skin is sizzling like bacon in a hot pan. Some women sweat profusely, others turn red, and still others feel a chill and have shivering afterward.

The intensity, frequency, and severity of hot flashes and night sweats is as individual and unique as each woman is. Not everyone is troubled by symptoms. There are women who barely notice any change at all, sailing right through, wondering what all the rest of us are whining about. However, there are enough of us who do have such severe, intense, thunderstorm-like hot flash and night sweat activity that we'll do anything to feel better.

Not everyone has severe hot flashes and night sweats. Instead, some women will experience different symptoms, such as shivering and chills, which aren't as common in menopause and rarely mentioned as a symptom. Other women will have painful muscle aches and more fatigue, which are easily mistaken for other conditions. These less common symptoms often lead women to wonder if they're normal and their healthcare providers to order expensive medical tests

Other women will not notice any flashes of warmth, but will feel as if their hearts are beating out of control, which is very scary. Some researchers believe that this is a result of the "fight or flight" response that is triggered by the fluctuations in neurotransmitters, which can lead to hot flashes in some women. Sleep disturbances are also a symptom of menopause that many people chalk up to night sweats. However, sleep issues may stem from other causes, such as restless leg syndrome or needing to go to the bathroom frequently. No matter what the cause, lack of sleep inevitably leads to many issues that negatively affect the quality of our lives and the lives of everyone around us. Besides the fatigue that creeps up and causes women to want to nap and go to bed at 7 PM, loss of sleep impacts mood, relationships, and concentration. It's widely known that when people are deprived of sleep they become more irritable, are forgetful, and are more prone to a variety of illnesses. Many women say that they suddenly have trouble finding the right word or keeping track of simple things like birthdays or getting things crossed off their to-do lists. With sleep deprivation, relationships are affected by a much shorter fuse and an irritability that may feel raw, like an itchy rash that makes it nearly impossible to stay on an even keel and not react in anger to minor frustrations.

I want you to know that you will make it through this part of your journey. Even if you have horrible symptoms, you don't have to resort to crazy, unproven treatments to feel like yourself again. There are safe and proven options to fit anyone's lifestyle that range from doing nothing and letting the symptoms pass to using prescription medications and hormones.

I also want you to know that the journey through menopause will transform you into someone who is stronger and wiser than ever before. When it comes to happier and healthier, that's highly likely if you follow the tips sprinkled throughout this book.

When it comes to hot flashes, night sweats, and other menopausal symptoms, no two women are alike. However, you may recognize some of your own experiences in what Mary, Lora, and Lynn faced during their menopausal transition.

MARY'S STORY

Mary woke up drenched for the fifth time that night. She was so exhausted that she didn't have the energy to be as angry as she would have been under normal circumstances. The pillow was wet behind her head, her nightgown was clinging to her, and she felt clammy. Besides that, she had to pee, again. As she explained to me during one of our regular walks, it seemed that within weeks of her fiftieth birthday bash, she plunged into the steaming cauldron of menopause. "The Menopause Fifty Fairy showed up," she said. "She waved her wand, and then presto, change-o, I'm having seven to ten night sweats every night and a half a dozen hot flashes every day. This sucks!"

"Irritable, too?" I ventured carefully.

"Oh, yeah, watch out," she said. *"I had no warning, no hint that this was coming. My periods are mostly regular, you know, every six to eight weeks, skipping now and then and when they do come, they're a little heavier. These sweats are doing me in. I'm exhausted, my memory is shot, and I just want to step into the freezer to cool off."* She went on to describe how her hot flashes were like a wildfire bursting throughout her body, triggering a racing heart.

Initially, she thought she was having a heart attack because of the roaring in her ears, but since she had no chest pain and the feeling went away abruptly, she dismissed it as part and parcel of her hot flashes. Not only did she have tiny beads of sweat on her forehead, but she also felt as if a waterfall was gushing from her underarms.

Mary's under-eye circles weren't just dark; they were black holes. Normally her infinite patience and sense of humor could diffuse any tense situation, but now with her lack of sleep, she had become a self-described *"bitch,"* snapping at every little thing. Mary sighed when I mentioned that depriving someone of sleep was one of the main tactics used to torture people. *"Oh, that actually makes me feel better,"* she said. *"I thought I was going crazy. I just need some sleep, but I can't with these night sweats."*

We talked about the gamut of remedies that are available to treat hot flashes and night sweats. Mary didn't relish the idea of taking medication. As bad as she felt, she wanted to wait out this phase. When I mentioned that research showed that yoga breathing, acupuncture, and increasing soy in the diet helped many women, Mary perked up. Within twelve weeks of starting acupuncture, yoga, and drinking soy milk twice each day, her hot flashes decreased from six to eight each day to only three, which were much more manageable. The night sweats weren't as intense or as frequent, and soon she was sleeping soundly for four-hour stretches.

LORA'S STORY

Running to catch a plane was Lora's most frequent aerobic activity. She was on the road traveling at least two days each week. With regular meetings with clients only a short plane ride away, she was the embodiment of a frequent flyer. Though she tried to work in time to exercise at the airport hotels, by the time her meetings were over and the requisite business dinner paid for, all she wanted to do was unwind and check emails before collapsing into bed. When her feelings of warmth first started four months earlier, she thought the hotel thermostats might have been set too high and that she was using too many blankets. Then she noticed that her nightgowns and pillowcases were moist in the morning. All of these clues pointed toward the beginning of menopause, a direction she wasn't ready for.

Lora also noticed that hot showers and hot coffee in the morning started a series of searing hot flashes that left her drenched in sweat and needing another cold shower.

She began taking cooler showers and switched to iced coffee. Before long, it seemed to Lora that anything could trigger a hot flash, from the slightly anxious feeling she had when the security lines at the airport were too long, to seeing an email from her boss. Anything that sparked even a miniscule amount of stress could set off a major catastrophe of sweat that ruined blouse after blouse.

Lora resorted to stuffing tissue under her arms to keep from sweating through her clothes. She came to see me for relief, announcing, "I can't function like this. Just give me something, anything, to make these go away." Lora's periods were sporadic, appearing every two to three months, which meant that she was in the midst of perimenopause. After an exam, and reviewing all of the options that began with doing nothing and continued to trying prescription medications and hormones, Lora decided to start using hormonal patches. She acknowledged that there were risks and no free lunch.

As she said, "I need to function now, and I'll trade that for possible, remote risks later on." Because she was in good general health, had a normal blood pressure, no risk factors for cardiovascular disease, and no family history of breast cancer, she was a good candidate for any number of options, including hormones.

We discussed the risks and benefits of using hormone treatment (see Chapter 10). Lora decided to use an estrogen patch and take Prometrium, oral micronized progesterone. She called two weeks later. She was finally sleeping through the night for the first time in months and rarely had a hot flash. She felt as if she had her life back. The following year, when she came in for her annual, we reviewed the latest research, and she decided that since she wasn't having any side effects, she would continue using hormones.

LYNN'S STORY

Lynn loved plants and worked part-time at a local nursery when she wasn't tending to her own large vegetable patch or volunteering in the community garden near her house. Working outside most of the day, watching the plants grow in the hot sunshine, was something she had always enjoyed. However, over the last few months she found the midday heat intolerable. Waves of hot flashes and a racing heart made it difficult to concentrate. She raced to finish as much weeding, watering, and pruning as she could during the cooler early morning hours.

Lynn slept soundly; she always felt a sort of "happy tired" at the end of a productive day and fell asleep within minutes of her head hitting the pillow. If she had night sweats, she never noticed, but then again, she was able to sleep through just about anything, including her husband's bear-like snoring. All that changed with the onset of her hot flashes. Several times each night, the back of her neck was drenched in sweat. Her pillowcases were clammy, and she needed at least twenty to sixty minutes to fall back to sleep.

Lynn's hot flashes sapped all of her energy during the day, and the frequent waking at night left her drained. She resorted to lugging a cooler filled with icepacks and cold water to the garden each day. Throughout the day, she'd swig on the water and stuff icepacks under her shirt or wrap them around her neck to cool off. She often ran the garden hose over her wrists just to get some relief.

Lynn's periods had stopped abruptly about fifteen months earlier. She kept hoping her hot flashes would dissipate in the fall and winter with cooler weather, but when there was no sign of that, Lynn tried black cohosh, a medicinal herb she had heard might help with her symptoms. There was some improvement for a few months, but then the hot flashes got worse again. She visited an acupuncturist on the advice of one of her gardening friends. The customized herb mixture that the acupuncturist gave her to get her qi ("chi"), or essential life force, in alignment tasted awful, yet they did work to reduce the number of hot flashes and night wakenings by about a third. She was so desperate for relief, she took the tablets without knowing what they contained because the ingredients were listed in Chinese. Although she had never heard of most of the herbs and other ingredients in the mixture, she figured they were natural and so must be safe. She was willing to try anything to get her life back.

Lynn also tried slow, deep breaths every morning and as soon as she felt a hot flash start. The breathing exercises helped her feel calmer, but she wanted to get the hot flashes under better control and was desperate for some help in sleeping through the night.

Lynn came to see me to ask for prescription sleeping pills. As we talked about the underlying cause, it was clear that her symptoms were related to menopause. Lynn was adamant that she wasn't interested in any hormone treatment but was open to the idea of using prescription antidepressants to help her manage her symptoms and get more sleep at night. Several of her friends were on antidepressants and didn't seem to be having any unusual side effects. I explained that many of these medications did not have FDA approval for the treatment of hot flashes and night sweats, but that many women found improvement in their symptoms. Lynn decided to give them a try for a few months. She was especially interested because there were no reported risks of blood clots, heart disease, or breast cancer with antidepressants.

I advised Lynn that she might not see much improvement for the first three weeks. A month later, when I checked in with her, she reported that she was finally getting six to eight hours of sleep each night and felt more energetic and like herself. She found that her irritability was declining in step with the reduction in the number and severity of hot flashes she had throughout the day and night. The best part was that she was able to work in the garden more without feeling completely drained. Recently Lynn came in and was happy to learn that an antidepressant—paroxetine (brand name Brisdelle)—had been approved by the FDA as the first nonhormonal remedy for hot flashes and night sweats. This medication, paroxetine, which is also marketed as Paxil, has been used for many years to treat depression and anxiety. When women who took Paxil also reported that *they had fewer hot flashes and night sweats, more studies were done that confirmed the beneficial effects on menopausal symptoms, which led the FDA to approve a lower dose of paroxetine (Brisdelle) to treat hot flashes and night sweats.*

Because she felt so much better, Lynn referred her friend, Sandi, to see me. Sandi had been diagnosed with breast cancer five years previously. She was told by her oncologist that hormones were out of the question, but she still wanted to discuss other options to help with the night sweats that were plaguing her. I recommended she try the nonhormonal prescription medication gabapentin before bed. Besides helping to improve temperature regulation, it also helps women sleep. Though gabapentin is not approved by the FDA to reduce hot flashes and night sweats, it works for these symptoms. Many healthcare providers have recommended it for years to women who are breast cancer survivors because it works well without the risk of taking hormones. I don't usually recommend it for daytime use, as the most common side effect is drowsiness.

Lynn found relief from using an antidepressant, and Sandi felt better using gabapentin. Both women told me that not worrying about serious side effects from using hormones was also a huge relief.

THE NITTY-GRITTY ON HOT FLASHES AND NIGHT SWEATS

In order to fully comprehend why certain remedies work for hot flashes and night sweats, it's helpful to understand the biology that influences all of the various physical symptoms and changes you may be noticing. The first step in understanding is to agree upon the definitions of the four phases of menopause. These include premenopause, perimenopause, menopause, and postmenopause. Let's take a look at each.

- **PREMENOPAUSE**—Premenopause is the time when periods are regular and predictable, with no symptoms of hot flashes, night sweats, or vaginal dryness. Hormone levels vary during the menstrual cycle but are within a normal range. The cycles are in balance. This phase begins in the teens and continues until the periods start to become irregular. Most women will reside in this phase until their late forties to early fifties.

- **PERIMENOPAUSE**—This is the time of transition between premeno-pause and menopause, when hormone levels start to decline and may also fluctuate wildly. This unpredictable and often wild "hormonal roller-coaster ride" occurs during the juncture between having regular, predictable periods and the time when periods stop completely. Peri-menopause is a challenging stage with hormonal upheavals and the possibility of wildly unpredictable periods. Many women skip several months without a period then have a phase of regular periods, then irregular periods. Any and every combination of skipping periods, heavy periods, and irregularity is common during perimenopause.

- **MENOPAUSE**—Surprisingly, menopause actually lasts only one day. What? Menopause occurs on the day when a woman hasn't had a period in one full year. Before that day, she's perimenopausal, and after she's postmenopausal. For the sake of consistency, however, we'll talk about menopause as more than one day and the time when a woman's body is experiencing a wide range of symptoms from barely any to life-altering transformations.

- **POSTMENOPAUSE**—This technically starts the day after menopause, when there hasn't been a period for one year plus one day. It occurs when hormone levels have declined to a steady level. Women may continue to have symptoms of hot flashes and night sweats, but they are usually not as frequent or intense as they were during peri-menopause and menopausal transitions. Women can expect to live a full one-third of their life, which is about thirty to forty or more years, after menopause.

Cooling-Off Cascade

This is going to sound crazy, but in menopause a hot flash is really our body's mixed-up attempt at cooling off. Really! The exact mechanism for how hot flashes occur is not completely understood. However, we do know that during a hot flash, there is rapid dilation of the smallest blood vessels in the skin leading to increased blood flow near the surface of the skin, which results in feeling rapid and overwhelming warmth. Hot flashes and night sweats are a crazy paradox. Never doubt the power of hormones—especially the absence of hormones to screw things up! In this case, the declining estrogen levels in perimenopause and menopause wreak havoc on our internal thermostat. The way that our brains regulate temperature, from shivering to sweating, transforms overnight.

Something as innocuous as taking a hot shower triggers the brain to perceive a slight temperature change. The brain thinks that it's too warm and initiates a cooling-off cascade of events, which has the exact *opposite* effect. We end up feeling warmer, not cooler. Prior to menopause, the brain ignores slight variations in temperature. A cup of hot coffee, a warm, cozy sweater, or a little nervousness doesn't affect us. But in menopause, all that changes. Now, the brain is literally sweating the small stuff.

Researchers believe that as estrogen levels decline, certain neurotransmitters, such as norepinephrine and serotonin, are released with stress or slight temperature changes. These neurotransmitters travel to a very confused thermostat, which overreacts and, in panic mode, goes overboard, sparking a rapid response to "cool off quick."

The cooling-off cascade begins with blood vessels near the surface of the skin quickly dilating to rapidly cool the blood. Sweat glands are also simultaneously activated to help dissipate the heat. Just to help things move faster, the brain tells the heart to speed up a little. Women may perceive a racing heartbeat and a rushing or roaring in their ears. So, in addition to a flush or flash of intense heat, possibly followed by sweating and shivering, a woman's heart may be racing and she may feel out of breath. These symptoms often trigger more stress and another hot flash can start up.

Dr. Robert Freedman, an internationally recognized expert in hot flash physiology from Wayne State University, has been studying what triggers hot flashes and how they occur. In his lab, he found that women can experience a hot flash with as little as a 0.05-degree change in their temperature.

That means that getting into a car that's been baking in the sun can cause a hot flash. Drinking hot coffee can lead to sweating through twelve-hour deodorant in five seconds. It also means that relaxing in a hot bath or taking a hot shower is out of the question. Women who smoke may also have more intense symptoms, as their blood vessels don't have the ability to dilate as quickly and diffuse some of the heat.

Recent evidence also shows that women who carry a few extra pounds of fat have more severe hot flashes and more in number. It's thought that the added fat has an insulating effect, which makes the body warmer to begin with. Women who exercise regularly and do weight training may have fewer and less severe hot flashes as their added lean muscle mass helps convert some of the other hormones that are stored in our fat to estrogen. This is another good reason to drop those extra pounds.

Over 80 percent of women will have hot flashes of varying degrees of intensity. It's not unusual for some women to experience hot flashes and night sweats for as long as five to ten years—or longer. The good news is that for the most part, over time, and we're talking months and years here, the intensity of hot flashes diminishes. Women with a history of breast cancer who are treated with tamoxifen, Evista, or aromatase inhibitors are more likely to have sudden and severe hot flashes and night sweats. These medications work to completely suppress and lower estrogen levels, leading to an instant menopause.

Understanding Hot Flashes and Night Sweats

You'd think with millions of women around the world suffering from hot flashes and night sweats, we would know exactly how they occur. Though there's a lot of research and conflicting ideas, one theory in particular makes sense to me. Using very elegant and well-designed studies, Dr. Robert Freedman came up with a theory of why women have hot flashes in menopause. He named this intricate biologic internal thermostat the thermoneutral zone (TNZ).

This temperature or thermoneutral zone is wide before menopause and narrows as estrogen levels decline. Prior to menopause, there can be large fluctuations in body temperature within the TNZ before the brain triggers sweating or shivering. After menopause, tiny temperature variations or even a hint of stress will start a cooling-off cascade resulting in shivering or sweating.

Dr. Freedman also found that:

- Women with no hot flashes have a wider TNZ than women with hot flashes.

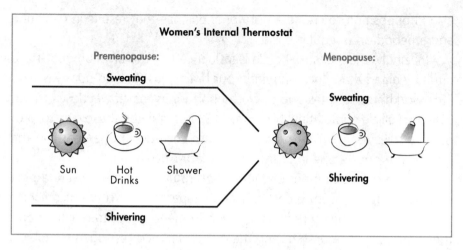

Figure 1. A woman's thermostat gets reset in menopause.

- A tiny rise in temperature, as little as 0.05 degrees C, leads to 70 percent of hot flashes in the lab.

- Estrogen levels aren't predictive of how wide the TNZ will be.

- Certain neurotransmitters and drugs, such as serotonin, norepinephrine, and gabapentin, influence the TNZ.

Why Estrogen Levels Disappear

Most, if not all of the symptoms associated with menopause, including hot flashes and night sweats, are related to estrogen disappearing into the sunset. This once plentiful hormone that was responsible for the changes that began in puberty, including our curves, breasts, and periods, begins to wane in the years before menopause.

Like most transitions, the decline in estrogen isn't always a smooth, predictable, orderly change but instead more resembles a roller-coaster ride, with wild fluctuations in hormone levels. To better understand what's going on, it's helpful to review the menstrual cycle.

Even as a menstrual period signals the end of the menstrual cycle, it also means that the process is starting back up again. The menstrual cycle is a fascinating and complex interplay of hormones working together and also in opposition to create a hormonal balance that results in ovulation and a period on a regular basis.

Amazingly, the menstrual cycle is influenced by the tiny kumquat-sized pituitary gland that's located within our brains, just behind our eyes. This little workhorse secretes two powerful hormones that travel down to our ovaries. Follicle-stimulating hormone (FSH) stimulates the ovary to produce follicles (eggs). These follicles in turn secrete estrogen early in the cycle and progesterone later in the cycle after ovulation.

Estrogen does a number of things that influence virtually every aspect of a woman's life, from breast size and shape and the curve of our hips to how long and heavy periods are, and in menopause, to our temperature control. Every month during the menstrual cycle, estrogen stimulates the lining of the uterus, also known as the endometrium, to grow and proliferate with blood and tissue to be ready for a pregnancy. If a pregnancy doesn't occur, this lining will be shed, which is what comes out with a menstrual period.

Luteinizing hormone (LH) helps the ovarian follicle mature and ovulate and then stimulates the secretion of progesterone. Progesterone is also responsible for keeping the estrogen levels and the growth of the endometrial lining of the uterus in check. You might say that progesterone is what balances the effects of estrogen in the uterus. This is an important point, because for women who have a uterus and who decide to use estrogen to help alleviate hot flashes and night sweats, progesterone will also be needed to help prevent the overgrowth of the uterine lining, which could lead to cancer.

Estrogen 101

In women, there are three types of estrogen produced: estradiol, estrone, and estriol.

ESTRADIOL OR E2 is the estrogen hormone we most commonly refer to when speaking about estrogen. Estradiol is present in various amounts at all times of our lives. It is the most potent estrogen.

ESTRONE OR E1 is considered a weaker estrogen and is the type of estrogen that is predominant in menopause. It is about one-tenth as potent as estradiol.

ESTRIOL OR E3 is the hormone that is increased during pregnancy. It is about one-eightieth as potent as estradiol.

For our discussion, I'll group them together and talk about estrogens as a class of hormones in general.

Estrogen's Effects

- Promotes breast development.
- Stimulates the lining of the uterus to grow.
- Promotes external and internal genital development.
- Maintains vaginal lubrication, pH, and elasticity.
- Reduces muscle mass.
- Increases fat deposition, especially around the hips and thighs.
- Helps maintain softer skin.
- Promotes optimal bone health by promoting bone building and reducing bone breakdown.
- Increases HDL cholesterol and triglycerides.
- Decreases LDL cholesterol.
- Increases pigment producing cells.

Progesterone

Progesterone exerts its influence on the lining of the uterus, stabilizing the growth and making it thicker with many more glands. In addition, progesterone prevents the unchecked growth and potential for abnormal growth that could occur with only estrogen's influence.

As the menstrual cycle starts again, the estrogen that revs back up helps the lining shed in a predictable, synchronous, orderly, and safe cascade, preventing hemorrhage.

So to sum up, in a normal menstrual cycle where ovulation occurs, there is more estrogen in the first half of the cycle and more progesterone in the second half. When ovulation doesn't occur, there's an imbalance of hormones, which can lead to irregular bleeding.

• •

Progesterone's Effects

- Keeps the uterine lining from growing out of control.

- Relaxes smooth muscle, including blood vessel walls, increasing the likelihood of varicose veins.

- Relaxes other muscles such as the bladder wall and the pelvic floor muscles.

- Slows down peristalsis in the intestine, which allows more water and nutrients to be absorbed, increasing the likelihood of constipation.

- May increase appetite.

- Influences mood.

• •

Why Do We Care About the Menstrual Cycle?

By the time a woman is in her late thirties, the number of ripe and ready follicles in each ovary has significantly declined. Some become more resistant to the siren song of FSH and need more and more coaxing to awaken and start pumping out estrogen.

As a result, FSH levels increase as the pituitary tries to induce those few remaining follicles to get into the game. Like a parent who has to shout louder to be heard over their teenager's music, the pituitary is literally screaming at the ovary, "Get to work."

Prior to menopause, a woman's FSH level may hover around 4 mIU/ml to 7 mIU/ml. Around perimenopause it may be 12 mIU/ml to 20 mIU/ml. After menopause, FSH can be 40 mIU/ml or much higher, as the pituitary pumps out FSH in the hopes of stimulating a follicle and increasing estrogen levels. Though it's tempting to consider testing FSH levels to determine if menopause is on its way, levels can fluctuate from day to day and month to month. If you are tempted to have FSH levels checked, don't rely on just one; get a few values over a few months. My advice is to use your symptoms as your guide. If you're over forty-five, having hot flashes and night sweats, your periods are irregular, and your vagina is a bit dry, chances are you're headed toward menopause and you can save a lot of money by not testing your FSH levels.

Fewer Eggs Means Less Estrogen

With fewer follicles available to pump out estrogen, there is less estrogen throughout the body, unpredictable ovulation, and less progesterone. As estrogen levels decline, women experience a variety of symptoms, including irregular periods and vaginal dryness, which may occur years before hot flashes and night sweats arrive.

By the time our periods stop altogether in menopause, the effects of less estrogen can be seen in how we look, how we feel, how much sleep we're getting, our moods, and whether we can concentrate. Below the surface, the lower levels of estrogen affect how thick our bones are, whether our vaginas are moist, our sex drive, and even our cholesterol levels.

HORMONE TESTS: ARE THEY HELPFUL?

Just as each woman's experience of menopause is as unique as she is, the hormone levels that correspond to symptoms are just as unique. Two women may have the same level of estrogen and have completely different symptoms. The amounts of estrogen circulating in our bodies haven't been shown to correlate with symptoms or the absence of symptoms. To the question, Are hormone tests helpful? The answer is no, they're not—at least not now, with our current understanding and level of sophistication with testing. It's more valuable to treat a woman based upon her symptoms.

Testing for FSH, estrogen, and progesterone levels is not recommended as these can vary from day to day and week to week and may not have any relationship with a woman's symptoms. Especially in perimenopause, when the values fluctuate from high-highs to low-lows, the testing can further confuse the strategy for treatment. After all, there are both hormonal and nonhormonal treatments available, which is why we base the treatment options on symptom relief, not on replacing a certain amount of hormones that are variable to begin with.

EXCEPTION: FOR WOMEN ON THE PILL. One exception to not testing for hormone levels is for women who are using the birth control pill to regulate periods and perimenopausal symptoms. In this case, taking the pill will mask any symptoms of menopause. If you or your healthcare provider is wondering if you're menopausal, simply stop taking the pill for one week. Then, after the week has passed, test your FSH level. By then the FSH suppressing effects of the pill will have dissipated, and you can get a better idea of what stage of menopause you might be in. This is recommended if a woman is considering going off the pill for side effects or when considering if it's time to switch to other remedies for symptoms.

EXCEPTION: IF THERE'S HEAVY, IRREGULAR BLEEDING. A second exception to not testing is in cases of women with heavy, irregular bleeding. Here, testing FSH levels can help determine where in the menopausal transition a woman is.

Salivary Testing

Testing the saliva for hormone levels has not been shown to be beneficial or reliable. The amounts of estrogen and other hormones in saliva vary throughout the day from one minute to the next. There's also never been a correlation between salivary levels of hormones and blood levels. It's impossible to use the values from salivary testing to determine much of anything. Further, normal values for hormone levels in saliva have never been established and verified by an independent lab. Therefore, I don't advise salivary testing and neither does the North American Menopause Society. Again, use your symptoms as your guide for treatment.

Hair Testing

Like salivary testing, testing hair for hormone levels has not been shown to be of any benefit. The amounts of hormones in the hair will vary depending upon the length of the individual strand and other factors, such as how fast the hair grows. Normal values also haven't been established; therefore, I don't advise that women use their hair to test hormone levels.

THYROID HORMONES AND CONCERNS

As we age, other hormone levels are also changing. Of all the hormones that influence a woman's life, the thyroid hormones are among the most important. Approximately 10 percent of women will develop a thyroid disorder during their lifetime, and many of these are discovered during menopause. Women with any type of thyroid disorder are also more likely to lose bone mass more rapidly, making it especially important to have bone mineral density testing regularly (see Chapter 14).

Thyroid hormones affect virtually every aspect of how our bodies function. It's important to have thyroid screening tests at menopause because many symptoms that we attribute to menopause could also be from an underperforming (hypo) or overperforming (hyper) thyroid gland. The tests that are usually ordered are a thyroid stimulating hormone (TSH) and a T4.

Located in the neck, the thyroid pumps out two hormones, T3 and T4. These influence:

- Temperature regulation
- Energy level
- Appetite and weight
- Skin and hair texture
- The menstrual cycle
- How fast or slow our hearts beat

Hypothyroidism

This is the most common type of thyroid disorder, affecting 90 percent of people with a thyroid condition. With hypothyroidism, the thyroid gland is underperforming. People who are hypothyroid may be chronically tired and have difficulty getting out of bed. They may find that their hair and nails are brittle and that their skin is dry. They may find it difficult to lose weight and have little to no energy to exercise. With hypothyroidism, the TSH is elevated because the thyroid needs high levels of stimulating hormone to pump out even a little hormone.

Hyperthyroidism

Hyperthyroidism occurs in about 10 percent of people with a thyroid condition. People who are hyperthyroid seem to be running on 100 cups of coffee. Their hearts may beat rapidly, they may have difficulty keeping weight on, and they may have diarrhea. They are extremely hyperkinetic and have difficulty falling asleep. Though it sounds like you'd get a lot done with hyperthyroidism, this is a dangerous condition and should be treated right away. With hyperthyroidism, the TSH will be low because the thyroid gland needs little stimulation to produce even modest amounts of hormone.

Signs of Hypothyroidism:

- Feeling tired with low energy all the time
- Slower metabolism
- Cold intolerance
- Weight gain or difficulty losing weight
- Hair loss and/or coarse, dry hair
- Depression
- Decreased sex drive
- Change in menstrual cycles

Signs of Hyperthyroidism:

- Palpitations
- Increased metabolism
- Heat intolerance
- Weight loss
- Warm, moist skin
- Nervousness and insomnia
- Breathlessness
- Change in menstrual cycles

Hashimoto's Thyroiditis

Hashimoto's thyroiditis is an autoimmune thyroid disorder that may be more difficult to detect. People with Hashimoto's thyroiditis may experience swings between having symptoms consistent with hypothyroidism and then having symptoms of being hyperthyroid. Although the TSH levels can be normal, people are very symptomatic, and the variation in symptoms and confusing lab results may lead to much frustration until the cause is identified. If you suspect that you have an underlying thyroid condition, ask your healthcare provider to go the extra step and test for the presence of thyroid antibodies in addition to checking the TSH and T4.

OTHER HORMONES THAT AFFECT MENOPAUSAL SYMPTOMS

There are many other hormones that influence menopausal symptoms, including DHEA and testosterone.

Dehydroepiandrosterone (DHEA)

DHEA is a hormone produced by the adrenal glands and is considered a precursor hormone for estrogens. As we age, DHEA levels drop. Supplementing with DHEA to help relieve menopausal symptoms is controversial, because DHEA can be converted or aromatized by fat into estrone and also into testosterone. Some healthcare providers recommend DHEA suppositories, though they are not FDA approved, as a treatment for the vulva and vagina to help with dryness. Although some European studies have shown benefit, others are inconclusive about the benefits. DHEA is available as a supplement in the United States and by prescription in Europe. There are reports of women with a history of breast cancer who are unable to use vaginal estrogen and find benefit from using vaginal DHEA.

Testosterone

Throughout our lives, our adrenal glands and ovaries produce small amounts of testosterone. Although testosterone is considered an "androgenic" or male-type hormone, women also have testosterone circulating in their body. Women with polycystic ovarian syndrome (PCOS) may have very high levels of testosterone, leading to deeper voices, loss of hair on their head, more acne, coarse facial hair, enlargement of the clitoris, and other "male-type" symptoms. Though there's a lot of individual variation, most women have lower circulating levels of testosterone than most men. Testosterone influences aggression, libido, and sex drive. As we go through menopause, these levels also decline.

Testosterone also affects cholesterol levels and may increase the risk of heart disease. Women who are considering testosterone should consult with their healthcare provider about the benefits and risks associated with its use. Right now, there is no FDA-approved testosterone available by prescription for use in women.

Nurse Barb's Tips to Figure Out
if You're in Menopause

You are premenopausal if:

- You're not using any hormonal contraception and your periods arrive within two to three days of when you expect them, which is the same as it's been for several years.

- The amount of flow with your periods is about the same as it's been.

- The amount of vaginal lubrication you have hasn't changed in years.

- In general, you sleep through the night without ever waking up feeling unusually warm, sweaty, or clammy.

- You can take a hot shower, hot tub, wear a few layers, and drink hot coffee without sweating.

- There's been little change in your sex life.

You might be perimenopausal if:

- Your periods are coming one to six weeks later than expected.

- The amount of flow with your period is much heavier or much lighter than expected.

- You've noticed a lot less vaginal lubrication than you've enjoyed in the past.

- You often wake up feeling warm in the middle of the night or have night sweats.

- You often feel warm or hot from triggers such as drinking wine, having hot coffee or tea, or from wearing multiple layers of clothing.

- Your sex drive is lower than usual or you have occasional, unexpected spikes of increased interest.

. . . .

You are menopausal if:

- You haven't had a period in twelve or more months.

- Your vagina feels smaller and dryer.

- Your sex drive has diminished.

- You have hot flashes and/or night sweats with certain triggers such as stress, slight temperature changes, and warm or hot showers.

. . . .

NEVER DOUBT THE POWER OF HORMONES

As you can see from this simplified explanation of a woman's biology during menopause, there are many hormonal changes that influence almost every aspect of our lives.

When our hot flashes and night sweats begin, it's just the tip of the iceberg in terms of the changes our bodies are experiencing below the surface. Estrogen, progesterone, and other hormones influence how much we sleep, whether we feel like we're on fire, our energy level, our moods, sex drive, periods, and so much more.

The decline in estrogen and loss of periods can be a welcome relief or a sudden storm that wreaks havoc in every aspect of life. Our biology is different from our friends, and yet there are some aspects to menopause that are universal. We know that as women age, the ovaries will not be able to produce as much estrogen as they did in the past. We also know that as estrogen levels diminish, profound changes will occur. While we can't turn back the clock, we can alleviate the symptoms and provide women options for relief.

7

Riding the Perimenopausal Roller Coaster

f it's not one thing, it's another! Irregular heavy periods are one of the most common reasons women seek care at menopause. As women hit their midforties, many notice that their periods arrive more frequently. Instead of every twenty-eight days, they may have a new period starting every twenty-one days. There may also be longer intervals of time between cycles that can range from five to sixteen weeks. It becomes impossible to predict when the next flow will start, and it may also involve a shocking amount of blood loss. Women may bleed heavily for one to seven days, and many describe passing very large, scary-looking clots.

Women describe themselves as feeling boggy and bloated. They may develop anemia and fatigue. Others, who've not been bothered by headaches, may suddenly start having migraines with their periods. Unpredictable cycles combined with experiences of heavy bleeding often lead to anxiety about having enough sanitary protection available, which can lead to women limiting their lives because of fears of accidents and leaking.

In normal cycles, there are four distinct phases:

1. **PREOVULATION**—More estrogen is produced, stimulating the growth of the lining of the uterus.

2. **OVULATION**—When the egg is released.

3. **POSTOVULATION**—More progesterone is produced, stabilizing the lining of the uterus.

4. **MENSTRUATION**—The levels of estrogen and progesterone both decrease rapidly, allowing for the synchronous and controlled shedding of the lining of the uterus—in other words, a period.

Irregular and heavy periods are often caused by ovaries that are not ovulating consistently and producing predictable, balanced amounts of estrogen and progesterone. Heavy bleeding may also be the result of polyps or fibroids.

Discussing heavy periods is one of the last taboo subjects that many women hesitate to bring up. Most women just put up with heavy bleeding and irregularity, believing that it's normal. For Krista, Jill, and Adrianna, heavy periods were indicative of other issues that needed to be evaluated and treated.

KRISTA'S STORY

Krista wasn't sure what to do next. She had been in the bathroom for thirty minutes and couldn't leave despite a looming conference call in fifteen minutes. She looked across the periwinkle blue tiles, toward the cabinet, trying to remember how many superpads she had left and whether it was enough to last through this afternoon's call.

Although her periods had been getting progressively heavier in the last few months, they had never been like this. She was worried about the amount of blood oozing out and was amazed in a detached sort of way at the size and number of clots she saw. She wondered if overlapping two superpads with wings would be enough to prevent ruining another pair of jeans.

Maybe if I'm lucky, I can run out to the drugstore and pick up more toilet paper and supplies, she thought. It was then that the thought of using diapers suddenly became at once both appealing and horrifying. This experience completely baffled her. Was this normal? Should she wait it out? What could this mean? What, if anything, could be done? She couldn't even leave the bathroom to go online to try to figure out what was going on.

What Krista didn't know was that she was on the hormonal rollercoaster ride of perimenopause and experiencing one of the least talked about and often the most troublesome symptoms—heavy and irregular bleeding. By the time she called me later, she was exhausted and desperate for answers. When I saw her the next day, we first did a pregnancy test, which was negative. I explained to Krista that unexpected pregnancy is still one of the most common reasons for irregular bleeding at midlife.

Krista's lab tests showed a very mild anemia and a FSH level of 18 mIU/ml, which meant that she could be perimenopausal. She had an ultrasound and a sonohysterography, which is an ultrasound during which a small amount of fluid is introduced into the uterus to separate the two sides of the uterine lining to better visualize any small polyps that may be lurking within the lining. Her ultrasound and sonohysterography were both normal. The next step was an endometrial biopsy to obtain a sample of the cells from the uterine lining to evaluate them for any abnormal growth.

All of these tests pointed to anovulation with an absence of progesterone's stabilizing influence on the uterine lining. Krista received an injection of progesterone and a prescription of Prometrium to take orally for the next fourteen days while we waited for the endometrial biopsy results. The results indicated that she had a benign, proliferative endometrium, which corresponded to our diagnosis of lack of ovulation (anovulation) and the absence of progesterone's stabilizing influence (which meant that she had unopposed estrogen) on the uterine lining. Krista's bleeding slowed down within days and completely stopped by day ten.

As this was her first episode of heavy bleeding, it was safe to take a watch, wait, and see what would happen in the next few months. Unfortunately, Krista's bleeding pattern continued every month for the next three months. After reviewing all of her options, she decided to use the Mirena intrauterine device (IUD), because it would deliver a consistent and small amount of progesterone to her uterus every day, decreasing the likelihood of irregular bleeding. She was also hoping that like many women who used Mirena, she wouldn't have any more periods. The insertion could be done in the office and only takes about two minutes, which meant that she could go right back to work that afternoon.

Krista had some slight spotting for the first three months after her Mirena insertion, then to her delight, her periods stopped completely and became a distant memory. Because she had no hot flashes or night sweats, and her FSH levels were consistently below 20 mIU/ml for several more years, she was considered perimenopausal.

JILL'S STORY

Jill had been putting up with "periods from hell" for years, just biding her time until menopause would put a stop to them once and for all. Lately, she was more worried about her lack of energy and the inconvenience in her busy schedule. At forty-nine, she was way past caring if she ever had another period again, having started at twelve and only having had breaks with her three pregnancies and while breast-feeding.

"I have a heavy period every four weeks like clockwork. The first day is usually heavy, and super tampons and overnight pads are fine as long as I change them every few hours. But for the last few months, I've had to change my pad and super tampon every hour, sometimes sooner. Now my period's heavy for three to five days, not for just a few hours. My periods still come when I expect them, but this amount can't be normal."

She was used to enduring a lot of discomfort without complaining or using medications and hadn't wanted to discuss heavy bleeding in the past, because she was worried that the only treatment would be a hysterectomy. Jill didn't want to end up like her mother, whose hysterectomy led to depression.

Jill's physical exam was normal, except for one thing. When she laid down flat on the exam table, she looked like a woman who was four months pregnant. "I can't seem to get rid of my potbelly. I know, it looks like I'm pregnant, right?" she asked. Jill wore tops that camouflaged her thicker middle and was trying to get out and walk with a friend a few times each week, but her potbelly stayed the same no matter how much she exercised.

When I examined her, I found a very large mass in her abdomen that extended to just below her belly button. It was hard and attached to her uterus. With a negative urine pregnancy test, it wasn't a pregnancy, and yet we would need to do an ultrasound to confirm my suspicions and rule out a long list of other possible causes. The ultrasound revealed a large melon-sized fibroid. It arose from within the muscle of the uterus and grew out into the abdomen. She also had two smaller fibroids, one of which extended to the lining of the uterus.

This could certainly explain the big tummy, but we needed to make sure there weren't any other causes compounding the problem. Jill's endometrial biopsy was normal, and her sonohysterography revealed several small polyps in her uterus.

After carefully reviewing her options, Jill decided that she would control her bleeding with a hysteroscopic removal of the polyps and the one fibroid that extended into the endometrial lining. The hysterocope is a small, thin instrument that uses a lighted camera to find and remove intrauterine polyps and small fibroids. This is a good option for women who want to preserve their uterus. However, Jill still had the problem of the very large, melon-sized fibroid. Not wanting to have a hysterectomy, she chose to have a uterine artery embolization (UAE) for the large melon-sized fibroid. With new, minimally invasive procedures, she had more options than her mother had had.

She was able to have both procedures on the same day with only epidural anesthesia and stayed in the hospital for two days, using a patient-controlled analgesia (PCA) to manage her pain. Her most annoying side effect was nausea and vomiting, which is common after an embolization. With a dose of Zofran, an antinausea medication used with patients who've had chemotherapy, she began to feel better within a few hours.

Jill was monitored with ultrasounds every three months after the embolization to see if the fibroid was shrinking. After fifteen months, it had regressed so much that she dropped two pant sizes. She still had periods every month like clockwork, but now that the polyps and fibroid were gone, they were more manageable and a lot lighter.

ADRIANNA'S STORY

Adrianna's irregular bleeding pattern was more worrisome than Krista's or Jill's—as she discovered in the most surprising place, her hair salon. Every six weeks she allowed herself one little indulgence, but that day she wasn't able to relax. Sitting in the black leather chair while getting her gray roots colored, she casually mentioned to her stylist that she'd been spotting almost every day for the last six months.

She was starting to worry. Only forty-two years old, and not having had any hot flashes or night sweats, she didn't think the constant spotting was related to menopause but didn't know what to do next. The stylist, who happened to be one of my patients, urged Adrianna to make an appointment right away.

Adrianna's periods had always been irregular. For her, skipping two or three months was typical. After high school, she even went a full year without a period, which was convenient as she was on the swim team in college. Once she started birth control pills, her periods became regular, and she assumed that everything was fine. Her periods weren't at the top of her mind until she tried to get pregnant. She and her husband tried for years. They were told by her doctor to keep trying, and she was told to lose weight.

Adrianna didn't know why it was so much harder for her to lose weight than her friends. At 5 feet, 4 inches and 170 pounds, she had been struggling with her weight since junior high. She could eat salads and baby carrots for a month, exercise two hours each day, and only drop a pound, while her friends could simply stop thinking about dessert and lose weight.

When she was trying to get pregnant, she had asked for hormone testing but had been given a prescription for Clomid (an ovulation-stimulating drug) instead. She became pregnant with twins after the third month on Clomid. After the babies were born, she was so busy that her irregular periods took a backseat to being a mom. Now she wondered if this continuous spotting was another sign that her body wasn't the same as everyone else's.

Adrianna's lab tests revealed several things. She had an elevated TSH of 12.5 ng/ml, meaning that she was hypothyroid. Her LH was 34 mIU/ml and her FSH was 13 mIU/ml. An ultrasound also showed more than ten small cysts in the right ovary and thirteen in the left ovary. Adrianna's cluster of symptoms, including her facial hair, acne, and the fact that she had multiple cysts in both ovaries, all indicated a diagnosis of polycystic ovarian syndrome (PCOS). This hormonal imbalance also meant that she was not ovulating regularly, which meant that she didn't have progesterone's limiting influence on her uterus and was at risk for endometrial overgrowth (hyperplasia) and cancerous cell growth in the uterus.

Her ultrasound also showed a slightly enlarged uterus with a very thick endometrial lining of 15mm. The endometrial biopsy confirmed my worst fears. The endometrial cells were cancerous. She had endometrioid adenocarcinoma. Adrianna was advised by two different gynecologic oncologists to have a complete abdominal hysterectomy with bilateral oophorectomy (removal of both ovaries). She would have her pelvic lymph nodes evaluated as well.

We started by immediately treating her hypothyroidism with thyroid replacement, as it would improve her body's ability to function at its optimum, especially prior to major surgery. Because women with PCOS are also at risk for insulin resistance and type 2 diabetes, I checked a fasting glucose, hemoglobin A1c, and a fasting lipid panel. Adrianna's fasting glucose was 86 and her hemoglobin A1c was 5.2, which meant that she was not a type 2 diabetic. Her total cholesterol was in the normal range, but her triglycerides were 220, which was an indirect marker of an underlying insulin resistance. We would work on this after getting her thyroid medications adjusted to see if it improved.

Luckily her cancer was caught at an early stage and only affected the endometrium and a tiny bit of the myometrium (muscle of the uterus). It didn't extend to her cervix or ovaries. She was a stage 1B, which meant that her prognosis was excellent. Nearly 90 percent of women with stage 1B endometrial cancer will be cured.

Adrianna's hair stylist told me later that she received a big bouquet of flowers from Adrianna for urging her to be evaluated. Her stylist's advice saved her life. With the removal of her ovaries, Adrianna's PCOS symptoms improved dramatically and she lost ten pounds. Her lipid profile also improved, but now she was having severe hot flashes. With her oncologist's consent, she decided to use an estrogen patch to treat her symptoms and to help protect her bones. Because she didn't have a uterus, she didn't need to add progesterone and could use estrogen alone.

THE NITTY-GRITTY OF PERIMENOPAUSE

Women are adaptable in so many ways, and it's no different when dealing with our periods. The truth is we have a lot going on and we're beyond busy. We just deal with heavy and irregular periods the best we can and hope that things will be better the next month.

Women put up with a lot of bleeding and discomfort before finally talking to their healthcare providers about the "periods from hell" that tend to surface during perimenopause.

Perimenopause is the ultimate roller coaster of hormonal shifts. Just like a real roller coaster, in perimenopause there are wild twists and turns, some predictable phases, and some unexpected free falls and jolting stops. In a way it's similar to puberty, where each woman receives a different ticket from her friends and family. Her ride has its own pattern, where anything can happen. Just when she's getting used to lighter or heavier flows, the roller coaster swerves into hot flashes and night sweats, and then drops into unbelievably erratic periods. Just as soon as one cycle is complete, the ride starts up again, but the next time around, anything goes. It's a brand-new pattern and may be completely different. The twists she's come to expect aren't the same because everything can change again without warning. No wonder women are drained and exhausted.

There's no reason to suffer and put up with the wild roller-coaster ride of perimenopause and heavy periods because the testing is easier and the treatments have evolved to be minimally invasive. All this adds up to women being able to get back to their lives faster than ever before.

To understand what's going on, it may be helpful to review what's normal first. For that, see Chapter 6. Whenever there's heavy bleeding, it's essential to determine the cause. There are many reasons why a woman approaching menopause might be having heavy bleeding. See "Some Causes of Heavy Bleeding" below.

Some Causes of Heavy Bleeding

- Pregnancy

- Fibroids

- Polycystic Ovarian Syndrome

- Hormonal imbalance

- Endometrial hyperplasia (precancerous, abnormal cell growth in the lining of the uterus)

- Anovulation

- Polyps

- Thyroid disorders

- Coagulation disorders

- Endometrial carcinoma (cancer in the lining of the uterus)

PERIODS FROM HELL

There are several reasons for "periods from hell." The most common is caused by ovaries that aren't ovulating regularly. In the years preceding menopause, the ovaries don't just stop producing eggs abruptly; instead, they sputter and wheeze, ovulating intermittently. Without consistent ovulation, the ovaries can't make enough progesterone to keep the uterine lining from growing out of control. This leads to a chaotic menstruation phase with uncontrolled, heavy bleeding (see Chapter 6). Absence of ovulation, or anovulation, is one cause. However, there are other reasons for irregular heavy periods around the time of menopause. The presence of polyps and fibroids in the uterus are also culprits that interfere with the uterus's ability to shed the lining in a controlled, synchronous manner, leading to heavy and irregular flows.

Polyps

Polyps are more common in women over forty. These abnormal growths have a skinny stalk that arises from the uterine lining. They can be as small as a grain of rice or as large as an orange. Polyps may appear singly or in clusters, causing irregular bleeding, spotting, and heavier periods. If left untreated, polyps have the potential to become cancerous.

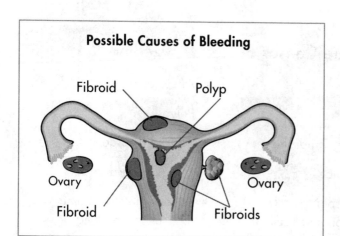

Possible Causes of Bleeding

Fibroid   Polyp

Ovary

Fibroid   Fibroids

Ovary

Figure 2.
A uterus with polyps and fibroids.

Fibroids

Many women are surprised to learn that up to one-third of women over age thirty have fibroids. They are typically benign, hard, noncancerous calcified growths. Fibroids can reside within the muscle of the uterus, impinge on the lining, or be attached via a stalk, like a large, hardened polyp. Large fibroids may press on the bladder, intestine, or other organs. My philosophy with fibroids is, "If it ain't broke, don't fix it." Unless the fibroids are growing rapidly, causing pain, or are so large that they interfere with your life or lifestyle, they don't need to be treated.

TESTING, TESTING, TESTING

The first step in an evaluation of abnormal bleeding is a complete history and physical exam. Then we can dive deeper into the possible causes of heavy bleeding, put on our CSI detective caps, get some lab tests, and review the various treatment options available. For all women with abnormal bleeding, these are the standard blood tests that most providers will request:

- **CBC—COMPLETE BLOOD COUNT.** This test checks for anemia that may result from too much blood loss. Within a CBC, we look at the hemoglobin level, which should be greater than 12 g/dL. Hemoglobin is a measure of the oxygen-carrying capacity of red blood cells. We're also interested in the hematocrit, which measures the percentage of blood cells within the blood. For women, it should be greater than 36 percent.

- **TSH—THYROID STIMULATING HORMONE.** The thyroid gland influences virtually every system of the body, including the menstrual cycle. Approximately 10 percent of women have a thyroid disorder. This highly sensitive test measures the amount of hormone that's needed to induce the thyroid to work. It shouldn't be too low and it shouldn't be too high. Like Goldilocks, a healthy thyroid needs just the right amount of stimulation from TSH to work properly (see Chapter 6).

- **URINE PREGNANCY TEST.** An often overlooked and common cause of irregular bleeding in perimenopause is pregnancy. Even when the odds of being pregnant are low, it's still important to make sure and get a urine pregnancy test. Women in their forties often assume that because periods are irregular that they can't become pregnant, however pregnancy can still occur.

- **FSH AND LH—FOLLICLE STIMULATING HORMONE AND LUTEINIZING HORMONE.** Though some providers would skip testing these because levels can vary from month to month, with heavy bleeding, testing can provide a snapshot of where a woman is in her journey through menopause (see Chapter 6). FSH is follicle-stimulating hormone and indicates whether the ovary is still able to produce eggs and estrogen. LH is luteinizing hormone and indicates whether the cycle is functioning as it should and there's adequate progesterone to balance estrogen.

If your provider does recommend FSH and LH levels because of heavy bleeding, the following values may help you determine whether you are still heading toward menopause, in the midst of it, or past it.

- **PREMENOPAUSE FSH.** FSH levels between 2 and 9 mIU/ml are consistent with a high probability of being able to ovulate and become pregnant. Levels of 10 to 15 mIU/ml, while still associated with regular periods, are often indicative of infertility and difficulty becoming pregnant.

- **PERIMENOPAUSE FSH.** FSH levels can range from 15 to 30 mIU/ml. As the number of available functioning follicles in the ovary decreases, the amount of FSH secreted by the pituitary gland increases.

- **MENOPAUSAL FSH.** A FSH over 40 mIU/ml is what's generally considered indicative of menopause. It's not unusual to see levels near 100 mIU/ml or higher.

- **LH.** The LH value is important as it relates to the FSH. This is a valuable test for women like Adrianna, with years of irregular cycles. Before menopause, if the LH is higher than the FSH, it may be a sign of polycystic ovarian syndrome (PCOS), which causes, among other things, infertility and irregular periods and puts women at high risk for endometrial hyperplasia and endometrial carcinoma, if they're not treated appropriately. For women with PCOS, the LH values will be two to three times the value of the FSH.

- **ESTRADIOL LEVEL.** Although there is much individual variation, and values do not always correlate with symptoms, estradiol levels sometimes help clinicians make sense of the entire picture. When a woman is in her twenties and thirties, her estradiol level can range from 25 to 75 pg/ml early in the cycle, increasing to over 200 pg/ml around ovulation. Many postmenopausal women who are not on hormones will have an estradiol level below 20 pg/ml. For menopausal women who are using estrogen, levels from 30 to 50 pg/ml are usually adequate to control symptoms. However, we rely on whether a woman's symptoms are adequately treated and not her estradiol levels to determine if her hormone treatments are effective or need to be adjusted.

- **PROLACTIN.** This hormone is secreted by the pituitary gland and is what induces the breasts to produce milk. Nursing mothers have high prolactin levels. Rarely, a prolactin-secreting tumor, known as an adenoma, can develop in the pituitary and interfere with normal cycles. A normal level falls below 24 ng/ml. For levels greater than 60, an MRI is necessary to rule out an adenoma. These types of tumors are almost always benign (noncancerous) and can be treated with oral medication (Dostinex) or with birth control pills.

- **ULTRASOUND.** An ultrasound is absolutely essential to evaluate heavy bleeding. It's important not to guess at the causes for bleeding, but to look at the size and shape of the uterus, the thickness of the endometrial lining, any uterine fibroids and polyps, ovarian masses and cysts, and other possible reasons for bleeding.

- **SONOHYSTEROGRAPHY.** This is a specialized type of ultrasound that can be done in a clinic or provider's office without anesthesia. A small, thin, flexible tube is passed into the uterus. Then a small amount of fluid is injected through the tube, which partially fills up the uterus and separates the sides, creating a better view of any abnormal structures, like fibroids or polyps that may arise from the lining.

- **ENDOMETRIAL BIOPSY (EMB).** This test should be offered to every woman with abnormal bleeding. It's easily done in a clinic or health-care provider's office. Often a local anesthetic is injected into the cervix to avoid discomfort and pain, and then a thin, flexible tube is passed through the cervix into the uterus. A small amount of suction is employed to remove some of the cells, blood, and tissue from the uterine lining. The endometrial cells are then examined by a pathologist for evidence of normal, abnormal, precancerous, or cancerous cells in the uterus.

Endometrial Biopsy Results

Normal Results

Atrophic	Unable to respond to hormonal stimulation
Proliferative	Preovulatory stage, estrogen dominant
Secretory	Postovulatory stage, progesterone dominant

Abnormal Results

Endometrial Hyperplasia	May progress to cancer if left untreated
Cystic Hyperplasia	Rarely progresses to cancer
Adenomatous Hyperplasia	10 percent will progress to cancer
Atypical Adenomatous Hyperplasia	25 to 50 percent will progress to cancer
Endometrioid Adenocarcinoma	Cancerous cells found

For more information on endometrial cancer, see the American Cancer Society's information at: www.cancer.org/Cancer/EndometrialCancer/index.

- **DILATION AND CURETTAGE (D&C).** In the past, this procedure was done more often as it was diagnostic and at the same time removed quite a bit of the lining that caused the problematic bleeding. This procedure is similar to an endometrial biopsy in that a tube is passed into the uterus and suction is used, but it is more extensive. With the advent of smaller, more efficient endometrial biopsy sampling tubes, D&Cs are used much less often and are not recommended. In a D&C, the lining of the uterus is scraped and more suction is applied to remove much more tissue and blood. A woman might be given conscious sedation through IV medication or this may be done under anesthesia.

- **HYSTEROSCOPY.** This test may be performed in a clinic, doctor's office, or outpatient surgery center so that local, regional, or general anesthesia can be used. Hysteroscopies can be used to both diagnose and treat fibroids and polyps within the uterus. A hysteroscope is a thin, flexible scope with a light and a camera that magnifies and projects what the practitioner is seeing onto a screen. This provides a close-up, magnified view of the inside of the uterus and the lining. Using very small instruments that are passed through the hysteroscope, polyps and fibroids can be removed.

- **OPTIONAL TESTS.** Blood tests for von Willebrand disease and other inherited blood coagulation disorders might be considered for any woman with a long history of excessive bleeding.

POLYCYSTIC OVARIAN SYNDROME AND IRREGULAR BLEEDING

For women like Adrianna, there's often a long history of irregular periods that put them at risk for more ominous consequences in midlife. Remember that estrogen causes proliferation or growth in the lining of the uterus, while progesterone causes the lining to become thicker, with more glands. We need both hormones for the lining to shed in a synchronous manner, without hemorrhage. We also need the balancing effects of progesterone to keep the estrogen from being too much of a good thing. When the uterine lining is only exposed to estrogen, and there is no progesterone, it may continue to proliferate and grow out of control. This situation is known as "unopposed estrogen."

When estrogen is unopposed, it can cause wild proliferation in the uterine lining without the limiting effects of progesterone. In rare cases, about 3 in 100, the cells will start to grow abnormally, becoming precancerous (hyperplastic) or worse, progress to cancer. This condition is more likely when a woman has polycystic ovarian syndrome (PCOS), which causes irregular periods and infertility. There isn't regular ovulation, which means that the lining of the uterus doesn't have the balancing effects of progesterone.

Had Adrianna's provider ordered some simple blood tests for FSH and LH and taken a peek at her ovaries prior to prescribing Clomid, they might have known that her years of irregular cycles were caused by PCOS, leaving Adrianna at risk for abnormal bleeding and worse, endometrial cancer.

Signs of Polycystic Ovarian Syndrome (PCOS)

- Absent or irregular periods
- Acne
- Increased hair growth on face and body
- Insulin resistance
- Difficulty losing weight
- Infertility

TREATMENTS FOR HEAVY BLEEDING

For all women with heavy bleeding, we need to first stop their bleeding and start them on supplemental iron to help mitigate the anemia they have or are at risk for. The lack of progesterone resulting from the absence of ovulation is the next thing to correct. Giving progesterone will stabilize the uterine lining and decrease the flow. This will often work, even if fibroids and/or polyps are contributing to the problem.

Fortunately, we have more choices now than our mothers and grand-mothers did for heavy bleeding. Unlike the past, when hysterectomy was the only solution, there are other effective options that every woman should consider.

Birth Control Pills

The first treatment most women try is using birth control pills with estrogen and progesterone to help counteract the imbalance of hor-mones that results when ovulation doesn't occur. Some women prefer to use the NuvaRing, a contraceptive ring that is inserted into the vagina. The NuvaRing contains the same estrogen and progesterone hormones as the pill; they are just absorbed through the vagina instead of the stomach as the birth control pill is. These not only prevent preg-nancy, they also reduce the amount of flow and the number of days of bleeding. Women who are nonsmokers are able to stay on low-dose birth control pills or the NuvaRing until their early fifties. Smokers, and especially smokers over thirty-five, have a ninefold increased risk of blood clots, which means that they should not be taking the pill or using the NuvaRing.

Mirena Progesterone-Containing IUD

Mirena is an IUD (intrauterine device) that has a tiny amount of proges-terone that is slowly released into the uterus over five years. Not only is this great birth control, with a better than 99 percent effectiveness rate, but it also helps reduce heavy menstrual bleeding. Mirena can be inserted during a routine office visit.

Endometrial Ablation

With endometrial ablation, only the lining of the uterus (endometrium) is removed, sparing the uterus. This is minimally invasive, since the pro-cedure is done through the vagina and cervix. There are different tech-niques that use heat, cold, or radio frequency to remove the lining. These procedures can be performed in an outpatient surgery center or a doctor's office. Endometrial ablation can be used for women with small fibroids that are less than 3 cm in size. This is a good option for women who do not want to have any more children as the ablation removes the lining of the uterus.

TREATMENT FOR FIBROIDS

Unless fibroids are affecting a woman's life or her lifestyle, by causing pain or pressure, it's perfectly reasonable to just monitor them every six months with pelvic exams and ultrasounds. However, if necessary, there are several treatment options for fibroids.

Myomectomy

This is a surgical removal of the fibroid while keeping the uterus intact. This is a minimally invasive surgical procedure that can be done in an outpatient surgery center. Women recover much faster when only the fibroid(s) are removed through the vagina using a hysteroscope or a laparoscope and hysteroscope at the same time. Depending upon the study that you read, the effectiveness of myomectomies ranges from 70 to 90 percent. Another option is to use robotic surgery with the da Vinci System, which uses five laparoscopes operated by one surgeon and 3-D cameras that magnify the area.

Some women with fibroids who decide to have a myomectomy are pretreated for several months with an injectable medication known as Lupron or Synarel, which shrinks the fibroid. These medications have some significant side effects, most notably hot flashes and night sweats.

Uterine Artery Embolization (UAE)

Also called uterine fibroid embolization (UFE), this is a noninvasive procedure in which a small incision is made in the groin to access the femoral artery. A catheter is then inserted into that artery and advanced up to the main uterine arteries, until the branch that supplies blood flow to the fibroid is located. Once there, small clotting particles are injected into the artery and the smaller arterioles that provide blood flow to the fibroid. The injected clot stops the blood flow to the fibroid, which, ulti- mately, over the course of several months, leads to shrinking. The clot doesn't move beyond the fibroid, and there's no risk of stroke or blood clots in other areas of the body. A UAE is approximately 90 percent effective.

Side effects include pain at the femoral artery site of catheter insertion. There's also the possibility of "postembolization syndrome." This after- effect of a UAE occurs as the blood flow to the fibroid is curtailed and an inflammatory process is triggered, leading to nausea, vomiting, fever, pain, and fatigue. These symptoms typically resolve on their own in a day or two.

Hysterectomy

There are over 600,000 hysterectomies done in the United States each year, with approximately one-third of them (between 150,000 and 200,000) performed for heavy bleeding. The other options listed earlier should be considered or tried first before resorting to major surgery.

A hysterectomy may sound simple in the descriptions below, but these only describe how they're done. And for years that's all that we, as healthcare practitioners, focused on. Now, however, we know that each woman will respond and adjust both physically and emotionally to the removal of one or more pelvic organs in her own way. There's a wide range of what's considered a normal emotional/psychological response to having a hysterectomy. Some women will be relieved and say "good riddance." Others will grieve the loss of the monthly reminder of their fertility and youth.

A six-week recovery means that a woman will be tired and unable to fully participate in her life. If there are complications, then she'll be dealing with added issues from the surgery. It's important to at least con- sider how the idea of having a hysterectomy might make you feel before you have one, and do talk to other women about their experiences.

Types of Hysterectomy

Only the uterus is removed in a hysterectomy. The cervix may be spared or removed at the same time. A hysterectosalpingo-oophorectomy means that the tubes and ovaries are also removed. Salpingo-oophorectomy is the removal of the fallopian tube (salpingectomy) and ovary (oophorectomy).

When both ovaries and tubes are removed, the procedure is called a bilateral salpingo-oophorectomy (BSO)—B (bilateral), S (salpinges or tubes), and O (ovaries).

All types of hysterectomy have the same list of possible complications, including infection, urinary incontinence, bladder and rectal prolapse through the vagina, fistulas, and pain.

- **ABDOMINAL HYSTERECTOMY.** Also known as an open hysterectomy, abdominal hysterectomy was the only way to remove the uterus until fifteen years ago. While other less invasive hysterectomies are increasing, the open hysterectomy still accounts for the majority of hysterectomies. This is considered a major surgical procedure, requiring general anesthesia and a hospital stay. For women with cancer, who need to have a complete visualization of the pelvis and removal of lymph nodes, the open approach is considered safer for improved long-term survival. However, robotic and other minimally invasive hysterectomies help women recover faster and are just as effective.

In an open hysterectomy, an incision between five and seven inches long is made in the abdomen, either along the bikini line from side to side, or up and down from the belly button to the top of the pubic area. The bladder, other pelvic structures including supporting ligaments, and intestines are moved out of the way, then the uterus alone or with the tubes and ovaries is removed. The skin, muscles, and other tissues are sewn back up, leaving a five- to seven-inch scar. After surgery, the woman will recover for a few days in the hospital and then needs at least six weeks to completely recover at home. The risks include infection, pain, urinary incontinence, bladder and rectal prolapse through the vagina, and fistulas. Though infections are rare, they can be prevented by using antibiotics both before and after a hysterectomy. Most women will need prescription pain medication after a hysterectomy for one or more weeks. More surgery may be recommended for incontinence, prolapse, and fistulas.

- **MINIMALLY INVASIVE PROCEDURE (MIP) FOR HYSTERECTOMY OR MIP HYSTERECTOMY.** Let's face it; having a uterus removed is invasive and major surgery that impacts a woman's life on many levels. All hysterectomies are invasive; however, there are some approaches that have fewer complications and are considered minimally invasive. MIPs are easier to recover from than an open hysterectomy.

    o **Vaginal hysterectomy**—Using the vagina as the entry point for the pelvis, an incision is made in the vagina to remove the uterus. The bladder, other pelvic structures including supporting ligaments, and intestines are moved out of the way. The top, back wall of vagina is then sewn up, leaving no visible scar. A vaginal hysterectomy means a shorter recovery and quicker return to normal activities. Because the incision is smaller and the approach is through the vagina, the area that can be visualized is smaller than what is seen through an open hysterectomy with an abdominal incision.

    o **Laparoscopic hysterectomy (LH)**—Several small one-quarter- to one-half-inch incisions are made in the abdomen. Then using one or more small lighted laparoscopes, which are telescoping instruments that house a camera and through which tiny instruments are inserted, the uterus is removed in small portions, while visualizing the procedure on a screen. Like other hysterectomies, the bladder, as well as other pelvic structures including supporting ligaments and intestines are moved out of the way. The small incisions in the abdomen are sewn up. The recovery for this type of hysterectomy is shorter than for an open hysterectomy.

    o **Laparoscopic-assisted vaginal hysterectomy (LAVH)**—This combines the benefits of the vaginal hysterectomy with the added visualization from a laparoscope in the abdomen. Several small one-quarter- to one-half-inch incisions are made in the abdomen. Then using one or more small, lighted laparoscopes, which are telescoping instruments that can house a camera and through which tiny instruments can be inserted, the surgeon can visualize the pelvis and move the bladder as well as other pelvic structures, including supporting ligaments and the intestines, out of the way.

The uterus is removed through the vagina. The small incisions in the abdomen and the top back wall of the vagina are also sewn up. The recovery for this type of hysterectomy is shorter than for an open hysterectomy.

o **Robot-assisted laparoscopic hysterectomy**—A newer method, called the da Vinci System, uses several (up to five) laparoscopes that are coordinated by one surgeon. The five laparoscopes are like tiny extensions of the surgeons hands and wrists that twist and turn in all directions, hold tissue, move it aside, and cut, all while the surgeon views everything on a magnified, three-dimensional screen. There is better visualization with the da Vinci System than with any other technique.

As with other procedures that utilize one or more laparoscopes, the surgeon can visualize the pelvis, but this time in three dimensions, and move the bladder and other pelvic structures out of the way—not just side to side but in all dimensions.

The tiny instruments within the laparoscope can be used to remove the uterus and other pelvic organs in small pieces so that a large incision isn't necessary. The uterus may also be removed through the vagina. The risks are the same as with other minimally invasive procedures.

Nurse Barb's Tips for Identifying Heavy Bleeding

When to contact a healthcare practitioner:

• You're soaking through a pad or tampon in less than one hour.

• You've been bleeding or spotting for more than ten days.

• You've had no period for twelve or more months, then you experience any bleeding or spotting.

. . . .

How much is too much?

Here are some guidelines to determine whether you're having too much bleeding:

- More than a total of 6 tablespoons or 90 mls for the entire period is considered excessive bleeding and needs to be evaluated.

- A regular tampon absorbs 2 to 3 teaspoons (10 to 15 mls).

- A superplus tampon absorbs between 3 and 4 teaspoons (15 and 20 mls).

- The average maxipad can absorb between 2 and 4 tablespoons (between 6 and 12 teaspoons or 30 and 60 mls).

- If you have any combination of soaked pads and/or tampons that adds up to more than 90 mls, then do contact your healthcare provider.

. . . .

TALK ABOUT YOUR PERIODS

Talk to your healthcare provider as soon as possible about any change in your periods. Let them know how often you need to change your pads, tampons, or both, and if they are adversely affecting your life or your lifestyle.

While the vast majority of heavy irregular periods are from an imbalance of hormones and can be easily treated, it's important to make sure the bleeding is not a sign of a more serious situation, including cancer. As you've learned, there are many more treatment options available now than ever before that are less invasive, less time-consuming, and fit into an active woman's life and lifestyle.

8

Staying Moist
South of the Border

One of the first signs that menopause is on its way, prior to any hint of hot flashes, night sweats, or troublesome periods, is that our vaginas, once as moist as a tropical rain forest, suddenly become as dry as the Sahara. Before you panic, let me reassure you that dryness isn't inevitable for every woman. A few lucky women are never troubled by any symptoms and barely notice any change. However, if you are one of the millions of women suffering from vaginal dryness, don't despair: there are safe and effective treatments.

If you are like many of my perimenopausal patients who grope around their nightstands for lubricant because their own natural slippery secretions are waning, you're not alone. In perimenopause, women may suddenly find that no matter how turned on they are, their lubrication faucet is turned off. At first, many assume that it's an isolated, one-time event, or that they weren't aroused enough. Then as this scenario repeats itself again and again, with lubricant becoming essential and not optional, women begin to face the facts. Their vajayjays are getting dryer and tighter.

Another startling side effect of declining estrogen levels is the discovery that our labias and vaginas are shrinking. One of my patients asked why her vagina was shrinking but not her waistline. Then she added, "Why didn't anyone tell me about this?"

At menopause and beyond, a woman's vagina gradually becomes smaller and less able to expand to accommodate a partner, a tampon, or even a finger. As she experiences more discomfort with sex, it's normal to tense and brace for the possibility of pain, further complicating matters by making any further relaxation, arousal, and orgasms virtually impossible. As menopause progresses and vaginal dryness worsens, many women find that intercourse is too painful to even contemplate. Unfortunately, some women give up on sex before finding out that they can restore their vaginal elasticity, moistness, and vitality and have a happier sex life.

If tightening and dryness weren't bad enough, itching, irritation, and an unpleasant odor often accompany the dryness. Declining estrogen levels are the culprit, causing thinning and more sensitivity. Perfumed soaps, wearing pads, and washing underwear in harsh laundry detergents may leave the labia and vulva irritated and inflamed. The genital skin is more vulnerable and less forgiving of friction, pressure, and tight clothes. Many women talk about having to drop their spin class and saying good-bye to wearing supertight jeans unless they want to suffer later with an ice pack wedged up against their private girl parts. *(Note to readers: Just in case you're wondering, the phrase: "private girl parts" is my term for the vulva, labia, mons, and vagina.)*

Still other women who haven't had a bladder infection in years will have symptoms of frequency, urgency, and burning with urination and develop more bladder and urinary tract infections. This is another consequence of declining estrogen levels in the entire genital region during menopause.

If vaginal dryness is left to its own devices, it only gets worse. This is one of the more insidious physical changes in menopause that doesn't reverse itself or improve over time. As women progress through menopause and beyond, this is one condition that should be addressed and treated, not only to prevent vaginal and bladder infections, but also for women who want to continue to have comfortable sex.

Although vaginal dryness and loss of elasticity don't occur overnight, by the time these changes register, these differences do seem abrupt. As you'll read in this chapter, prevention is key. We can keep the vagina, labia, and entire genital area healthy and vital by being proactive in our approach. Waiting until sex is impossible or for a serious urinary tract infection is too late. Providing treatment options at the very first signs of dryness is infinitely easier and healthier than waiting to try to regain lost ground once there's pain, infection, or the avoidance of sex.

I've been treating women with safe and effective treatments for years. There's absolutely no reason for any woman to suffer from dryness. Don't throw in the towel and don't give up. Although prevention is better, it's never too late to improve this condition.

A changing vagina is one aspect of menopause that affects virtually every woman, and yet few are comfortable discussing this aspect of their health with a provider. I'd like to introduce you to four women—Trisha, Kara, Bev, and Gina—who had a range of different experiences with their vaginal health. One or more of their stories may seem very familiar to you.

TRISHA'S STORY

Not every woman has difficulty with vaginal dryness during menopause. Trisha, a fun and vivacious fifty-three-year-old powerhouse was the exception to the rule. But was she really? She had four kids ranging from middle school to college and worked four days a week as a loan officer. She wanted to approach menopause naturally without using anything more than a healthy diet, one serving of soy each day, some exercise, and vitamins. Trisha blamed her four pregnancies, her desk job, and frequent business lunches for the extra twenty pounds she was carrying.

Even though her periods stopped two years earlier, Trisha rarely needed added lubrication during menopause and beyond. She was among a lucky group who continued to enjoy frequent, comfortable, satisfying sex regularly with her husband, Ben. Trisha lived by the adage: "Use it or lose it." She and Ben had sex at least one to two times each week, and she masturbated regularly to help her fall asleep.

There is a lot of wisdom to this approach. Regular sex and sexual stimulation promote blood flow to the genitals, keep the vaginal opening elastic, and can certainly infuse lots of feel-good neuroendocrine chemicals like oxytocin into a woman's system. No wonder Trisha was always smiling. For some women like Trisha, those extra pounds may be earning their keep, by producing a little added estrogen and increasing the levels just enough to help keep unwanted vaginal dryness at bay. That doesn't mean that women should gain weight to help with vaginal dryness, because added weight can increase hot flashes and night sweats by acting as a layer of insulation and increasing warmth.

As Trisha began a program to lose weight, her vagina stayed moist and healthy. It was also possible that as little as one daily serving of soy was providing just enough plant-based estrogens (phytoestrogens) to keep her vagina happy. It's impossible to know, but in any case, Trisha had a happy vagina. We should all be so lucky.

KARA'S STORY

Kara called me at the office in a panic late on a Wednesday afternoon. She was leaving on Saturday morning for a long-anticipated second honeymoon with Mark, her husband of twenty-five years and needed quick emergency advice. Her voice was breathless as she explained, "I was so busy taking care of my mother these last few months that I didn't get around to working on my own issues. I'm afraid it's going to be too little, too late."

Like many women in Kara's generation, she was balancing a full-time job, kids leaving home for college, and caring for her elderly mother. She was stretched thin from juggling too many demands, so much so that her needs weren't even on the never-ending to-do list. At her last annual exam eight months earlier, she had finally worked up enough nerve to mention to her doctor that she had been experiencing pain whenever she tried to have sex. No matter how relaxed and in the mood she was, her vagina was getting so dry and tight that she felt that things just weren't fitting together the way they had in the past. "We tried some lubricant, and it helped a little, but I felt like I was being ripped apart with a burning kind of pain, and so we stopped. It was scary, because in the moment I thought, I'll never be able to have sex again."

At her annual exam, her doctor had recommended vaginal estrogen cream for a few weeks, but when it didn't make any difference, she stopped using it. Then, as the other demands of her life took center stage, she found her interest in sex declining. She didn't think about her dryness again until a few months later, when she started looking for some bathing suits for her upcoming vacation. She and Mark tried to have sex again, but no matter how much she tried to relax and how much lubricant she slathered on the two of them, the feeling of being torn apart was too jarring, so they stopped. Casting about for a solution to her dryness, she decided to give the estrogen cream another try, but she stopped after reading the package insert and saw that breast cancer was listed as one of the possible side effects.

When I saw Kara in the office, she was worried. "I just feel lost. I'm going away to this great resort with palm trees and umbrella drinks—the whole picture-perfect vacation! We're both going to want to have sex, but what am I going to do? It's going to be a disaster unless you have a magic wand in your lab coat."

I didn't need a magic wand for Kara, but I knew that if I had seen her eight months earlier, this would be a very different kind of visit. At her annual exam, she had too much to do, too many things competing for her attention, and too little time to devote to her own body's changes. Plus, she didn't get the advice, instructions, or reassurance she needed. Kara was still having periods every four to six weeks and hadn't had any hot flashes or night sweats. That was reassuring. It meant that she was still producing a lot of her own estrogen. During her exam, I discovered that her vaginal dryness wasn't too severe.

I was confident we could help her have a great second honeymoon. She was interested in seeing what she looked like, so I handed her a mirror. Her vagina was only slightly dry. The labia were a tad smaller and a bit thinner. Though her vaginal opening was small when she was breathing normally and relaxed, it grew wider when I asked her to bear down as if she were having a bowel movement. Kara was astounded when she saw in the mirror how much her vagina expanded and opened up when she bore down.

After she saw how wide her vaginal opening became as she held her breath and pushed with her abdominal muscles, I asked her to try inserting a well-lubricated super tampon and see if there was any pain. Using the mirror, Kara found that by simply adjusting the angle and direction of the tampon there was a significant difference in whether she felt pain, resistance, or an uncomfortable sensation of stretching. Angling the tampon horizontally was painful, but when she angled the tampon toward her tailbone it slid right in without any pain. I showed her how to adjust the angle of her hips for sex by placing a pillow under her bottom and suggested a few alternative positions, such as lying on her side for more comfortable sex. That way, she could control the angle of intercourse, and with plenty of lubrication, sex could be pain free.

After her examination we talked about the benefits and risk of estrogen treatment in the vagina. I also gave her some samples of estrogen cream and some vaginal estrogen tablets, Vagifem, as well as an over-the-counter lubricant.

Kara was happy to hear that if she had an orgasm first through oral or manual stimulation, she'd be much more relaxed and receptive to intercourse. "That sounds like more fun," she quipped. Armed with more information, some samples, and my best wishes for a fun-filled second honeymoon, Kara was on her way after promising to call me with an update after her vacation.

Two weeks later Kara called with the good news that her sojourn to the beach was better than she expected. They had used up all the lubricant that she packed and resorted to using a little olive oil she ordered from room service. Not only was the sex fantastic, she found that pain wasn't an issue as long as they took their time, found the right angles, and lubed up. Things had been improving steadily after the vacation as the estrogen worked to help her vaginal tissue become more moist and elastic.

BEV'S STORY

I know that very few people are comfortable talking about sex, especially when they're sitting in a cold exam room and trying to keep a flimsy hospital gown from falling off. Whenever possible, I try to discuss these deeply personal issues with women while they are fully dressed. Bev, a technical writer who was working on her fourth science fiction novel, came in for her annual exam with no complaints. She deferred the pre-exam interview in the office since she was in a hurry. Her last period had occurred four months previously, and except for the occasional night sweat, she felt fine. When I asked her about sexual concerns, she just shrugged and said that everything was fine. Since she was in a hurry, I decided to complete her exam and then allow her to get dressed before asking more questions about sex. When it came time for her pelvic, I could see that she might be suffering silently and was perhaps too embarrassed to bring up the issue that was plaguing her private girl parts.

Bev's labia were getting smaller, and I could see evidence of a few hair-line tears around the vaginal opening. In the vagina, there were barely any of the accordion-like folds known as rugae left. The tissue of the vagina, which prior to menopause looks like multiple waves of soft ridges extending the length of the vagina, didn't have any of the ridges or rugae left but now was flat, smooth, and light pink. This happens as estrogen levels decline; the healthy, dark pink tissue becomes much lighter in color and loses its ability to stretch out like an accordion.

This was Bev's case, except for her vaginal opening, which was beet red. She also had a small amount of thin, gray discharge at the vaginal opening and coating the thin, smooth walls. I noticed a slight fishy odor. The redness indicated that there was some inflammation. I used a cotton swab to gently obtain a small sample of the discharge to check the pH and to examine the cells under the microscope.

The pH was over 5.5, so I had a good idea of what was going on. When I looked under the microscope, I kept searching in vain for any remaining healthy bacteria, known as lactobacilli, but there weren't any. What I did see were many clue cells that are indicative of an infection known as bacterial vaginosis.

When Bev got dressed, I met her in my office. She was surprised that the symptoms she had were caused by an infection. She thought that she'd just have to deal with discomfort, itching, and burning, and that somehow things would improve on their own. I asked Bev to start using Metrogel vaginal gel every night for five nights to treat her bacterial infection. We also talked about prevention. I gave her some samples of estrogen vaginal cream and Vagifem tablets to help restore her vaginal health and prevent recurrent infections.

After just a week, her vaginal infection had disappeared. Once she felt better again, she started using the estrogen cream every other night and found to her surprise that it wasn't as messy as she expected. The odor that she had been living with was also gone, and she found that she could wear her tight jeans without discomfort.

GINA'S STORY

Gina, a fifty-six-year-old accountant, who was a part-time yoga instructor on weekends, came to see me after a three-day holiday. She called the office for an emergency appointment. "I think I have a bladder infection," she said. "I haven't had one in years, so I'm not sure." Gina felt as if she had to urinate every five seconds, and although it wasn't the kind of thing she could ignore, she also dreaded the idea of going so often because it burned on the way out. She was puzzled because she hadn't had any symptoms like this in over twenty-five years.

As it turned out, the symptoms appeared as she and her husband were driving home from a romantic weekend away. Before this trip, they had enjoyed intercourse three to four times each year because her husband Joe's medications made it difficult for him to sustain an erection. They wanted to make this weekend special after seeing all those commercials on TV of happy couples holding hands in side-by-side bathtubs and thought, Why not? Let's go for it. With that in mind, Joe went to see his doctor for a prescription of Viagra.

It was a great weekend, with long leisurely lunches and a room at a romantic inn on the coast. On Saturday night, they skipped dinner and brought some bread, cheese, and champagne back to their room. Dessert was chocolate-dipped strawberries with a Viagra chaser. The sex was fun, though Gina was glad she remembered to slip a travel-size container of coconut oil lubricant into her makeup bag.

Monday night's drive home was a nightmare. They had had to stop at gas stations and fast food places every half-hour so she could use the not-so-nice restrooms. In one of the minimarts, she picked up some cranberry juice and sipped it all the way home. It was a long night with repeated trips to the bathroom.

When she came to the office, her urine dipstick test was positive, showing a small amount of blood, with many white blood cells. Luckily, she didn't show any signs of a kidney infection. During the pelvic exam, I saw the telltale signs of vaginal dryness. I knew she would be prone to more infections in the future if we didn't implement some preventive measures.

"You definitely have a bladder infection," I explained to Gina. "And *you'll need antibiotics to clear this up. We'll do a culture and sensitivity test, but it's most likely an opportunistic bacteria that hitched a ride on the love train this weekend and ended up in your urinary tract."*

I also provided Gina with samples and a prescription for Vagifem and estrogen cream to use on her labia to prevent future recurrences. Thankfully, her symptoms improved within twelve hours and were completely resolved in a few days. The vaginal dryness that kindled the fire took a little longer to treat, but after a few months, her dryness was under control. Gina and Joe were enjoying more frequent sex without frequent trips to the bathroom.

THE NITTY-GRITTY ON VAGINAL MOISTNESS

Sadly, stories of painful intercourse and vaginal problems are more typical than not. If I had a nickel for every woman who has approached me at a barbecue, bridal shower, or fund-raiser with this issue, I'd be on a beach in Hawaii with palm trees and umbrella drinks myself. I'm as frustrated as my patients that helpful information is hidden from too many women, and they struggle on their own searching for relief. Women who have painful intercourse are often told to use more lubrication, handed a prescription, but not given enough information to understand the warnings on the package or how to apply the treatments.

To make matters worse, no one tells them what to expect in the short and long term. The good news is that this situation can be remedied with safe and effective treatments that help restore the vagina to a healthy, moist, and happy state.

There are as many reasons for pain with intercourse as there are solutions. By far, the most common cause in the forties, fifties, and beyond is a result of declining estrogen levels, which leads to vaginal dryness, also known as vaginal atrophy. I really dislike the term *atrophy*. It implies a shriveled, dry, and withered appendage that is too far gone to nurture back to health; I prefer the word *dryness*.

Yes, the vajayjay does resemble the Sahara now more than the Amazon rain forest, yet vaginal dryness can be prevented and treated and not just for more comfortable sex, but for fewer bladder infections, less vaginal irritation, odor, and more comfort when sitting, walking, even sleeping.

Decline of Estrogen Levels

As estrogen levels decline, the process that started with puberty begins to rewind. Women like Kara begin to notice that their natural lubrication becomes less predictable. Women who could sense vaginal wetness just from having a sexually arousing thought or experience suddenly find that even with an orgasm their vagina just doesn't lubricate. Or they may have plenty of lubrication one day and scant the next. It can be confusing and frustrating at first, especially for women who are still having regular periods and who are years away from menopause.

Alterations in the vagina and vulva evolve slowly, years before the last period, but most women don't notice them until they have overt symptoms that can't be ignored. By the time a bladder or vaginal infection arrives, there's already been a long and slow reversal in vaginal health. Over time, the vagina's accordion-like folds, known as rugae, begin to flatten, thin out, and disappear, leading to loss of elasticity and the capacity to stretch. The vagina slowly loses it ability to widen and lengthen. Expansion and stretching can only go so far without the rugae's folds, which made the space wide enough to deliver a baby or long enough to contain a partner's penis.

The vaginal opening itself may become smaller, drier, and less pink, with a grayer appearance. If you were to look under a microscope at the vaginal cells, instead of being fluffy, flexible, resilient cells with lots of fluid, they appear constricted and compacted with a lot less intracellular fluid. Those cells comprise the vaginal mucosal tissue, which becomes paper thin, making it more likely to develop tiny microtears, which split the skin. This is not a pretty picture, and it hurts. Ouch!

Loss of Healthy Bacteria

In a healthy vagina, the mucosal cells produce glycogen, which helps nourish the healthy lactobacilli bacteria, which in turn keep the pH levels slightly acidic at 3.8–4.5.

With less estrogen, the way the cells function also changes. Production of glycogen decreases, which upsets the pH balance, making it more alkaline—greater than 5.0—leading to the departure of the lactobacilli.

Once the healthy lactobacilli pack up and leave, it opens the door for other problematic bacteria and yeast to take up residence. Many women develop a bothersome odor, itching and burning, dryness, and bladder infections as a result of the loss of estrogen that nourishes the lactobacilli in their vaginas, which are essential for vaginal health.

When the vagina starts losing its grip on estrogen and waves good-bye to the lactobacilli, thus becoming a shadow of its former self, it doesn't get better on its own. In fact, it always get worse, unless a woman has frequent sex or stimulation to increase blood flow to the area.

TABLE 8.1   TYPES OF VAGINAL INFECTIONS AND TREATMENTS

TYPE OF INFECTION	PH	ODOR	SEXUALLY TRANSMITTED	TREATMENTS
Yeast	<4.5	None or yeasty	No	**Creams, Gels, and Inserts:** Femstat, Gyne-Lotrimin, Gynezol, Monistat, Mycelex, Terazol, Vagistat-1 **Oral Medication:** Diflucan
Bacterial Vaginosis	>5.0	None or fishy	No; May be facilitated by sex	**Creams, Gels, and Inserts:** Cleocin (clindamycin), Flagyl (metronidazole) **Oral Medications:** Cleocin (clindamycin), Flagyl (metronidazole)
Trichomoniasis	>5.0	Fishy	Yes	**Oral Medication:** Flagyl (metronidazole), Tindamax (tinidazole)

Bladder Infections

You know the old song: "The thighbone's connected to the knee bone, the knee bone's connected to the shin bone . . . " and so on? Well, it's similar with the vagina, vulva, and urinary tract. The decline of estrogen prior to and during menopause affects the entire genital region and the urethra. With the vaginal opening and the urethral opening positioned right on top of each other, and both enveloped by the labia, they share lots of bacteria. As the pH becomes more alkaline with the loss of estrogen, the beneficial lactobacilli bacteria disappear, leading to an overgrowth of other more bothersome bacteria that can cause infections. We also can't forget that the rectal opening isn't too far away, with its colonies of bacteria that love to migrate toward the vagina and urethra. Add to that slightly weaker muscle tone, which means the force of urination may not be as strong, and you have a not-so-perfect recipe for frequent bladder infections.

Bladder infections are treated with antibiotics for three to seven days. There are a variety of over-the-counter and prescription medications that can also help alleviate the symptoms of burning and urgency.

Signs of a Bladder Infection

- Burning with urination
- Feeling that you have to go constantly
- A feeling of urgency, that you can't wait
- Urinating a small amount

Signs of a Kidney Infection

- Chills, nausea, vomiting
- Blood in the urine
- Low-grade fever
- Flank pain—back pain below the ribs
- Loss of appetite

TREATMENTS FOR VAGINAL DRYNESS

Several options are available to treat vaginal dryness. One of the most effective is the use-it-or-lose-it strategy, which helps maintain blood flow to the area, which in turn keeps the tissue healthy. For many women who find that sex becomes quite painful during and after menopause as estrogen levels decline, here are some other remedies to consider if you're experiencing discomfort, dryness, or pain with sex.

Nonhormonal Vaginal Remoisturizers

Many women have so much dryness that even wearing their own underwear is irritating. Other women find that something as gentle as wiping with toilet paper is painful. If there is leakage that comes into contact with vulvar skin, the irritation becomes much worse.

Women who are breast or ovarian cancer survivors, women on chemotherapy or aromatase inhibitors, and women who have had a hysterectomy with a rapid loss of hormones may experience intense dryness and may have been advised not to use estrogen. For these women and for women who aren't interested in using vaginal estrogen, the key is to keep the vagina as moist as possible and to help foster the growth of beneficial lactobacilli bacteria.

There are a number of over-the-counter, nonprescription, nonhormonal remedies for vaginal dryness. These are available online and through specialty pharmacies. They are pH neutral and provide a little moisture that is similar to what our own bodies make. These are *not* lubricants to be used with sex, although using them regularly can make sex more comfortable.

Although there's minimum research that supports the use of soy to help with vaginal dryness, because it contains plant-based estrogens, or phytoestrogens, many women find that eating one to two servings of soy goes a long way in helping relieve vaginal symptoms. Soy may also help with hot flashes and night sweats.

Over-the-Counter Remedies for Vaginal Dryness

Vaginal Remoisturizers

- Replens
- K-Y Silkie
- Yes lubricant
- Gyne-Moistrin

Vaginal pH Restoration

- RepHresh

Estrogen Treatment for Vaginal Dryness

The benefit of estrogen treatment for vaginal dryness at menopause takes time. The process that caused vaginal dryness occurred over many months to years. Although it would be nice if the treatment worked immediately, it takes at least six weeks for the estrogen receptors to completely reengage and another six weeks for the vaginal and vulvar cells to begin producing glycogen, inviting lactobacilli back and maintaining a slightly acidic pH. Most women will have a noticeable improvement in symptoms within a few weeks and feel better; however, it's important to have realistic expectations.

Topical estrogen treatment will not restore the vulva and vagina to what it was in the twenties and thirties, but using it can induce significant improvement, which can lead to less pain, decreased risk of recurrent infections, and more enjoyable sex.

Understanding the Risks of Estrogen Treatment for Vaginal Dryness

In terms of risk, there seems to be a big difference between using a small dose of estrogen in one localized area like the vagina, and using higher doses to treat hot flashes and night sweats with oral tablets, skin patches, topical gels, and creams that circulate throughout the body.

None of the serious side effects associated with hormone treatments for hot flashes has been associated the smaller doses of vaginal estrogen. It's also reassuring that when we look at retrospective studies, there doesn't seem to be any association between vaginal preparations and increased risk of breast cancer or of any other serious side effect.

Another encouraging aspect to the use of vaginal estrogen preparations is that the amount of estrogen used is significantly less than the amounts used to prevent hot flashes and night sweats. So little is needed that vaginal estrogen preparations don't stimulate the lining of the uterus to grow and thus don't need to be balanced with progesterone to prevent overgrowth, bleeding, or abnormal cell growth.

Putting the Risk into Context

It's very confusing to be reassured in a provider's office that a prescription for a vaginal cream, like Premarin, Estrace, the Vagifem vaginal tablets, or the vaginal ring, Estring, carries little risk, when the package insert says otherwise. All estrogens, whether they are oral tablets, patches, gels, or vaginal preparations are considered by the Food and Drug Administration

(FDA) to be in the same class of medication, and therefore, they theoretically carry the same risks. Right now, the FDA mandates that all medications within the same class carry the same warnings, even if the mode of delivery and the amount changes the risk compared to another mode of delivery or dose. With any estrogen prescription, all of the risks you see published are related to the Women's Health Initiative study (WHI) that was published in 2002 and are not a result of current research.

As I explain to my patients, while we can't guarantee that using vaginal estrogen is completely risk free, on the other hand we aren't seeing any study findings that demonstrate that using localized estrogen in the vagina is associated with any increased risks of breast cancer, stroke, heart disease, or blood clots.

Using Estrogen in the Vagina

There are three ways to reintroduce estrogen to the vagina. These are the FDA-approved hormonal treatments that are available only with a prescription.

- **ESTROGEN CREAMS.** Premarin and Estrace are the two vaginal estrogen creams available. They both come with an applicator that twists onto a tube of cream. The dose and amount of cream that's used can be adjusted depending upon your own healthcare provider's recommendations. I usually ask my patients to start with 2 grams every other day for two weeks, then to use 2 grams twice weekly. For women who are using Estring or Vagifem, I also prescribe some cream so that they can rub in a small pea-sized dab to the outside of the labia and around the vaginal opening for the first two weeks. It's like watering a very thirsty plant, most of the water goes toward the roots, and some is misted on the leaves. Using both often means faster relief.

- **ESTRING.** This is a small, flexible ring that is embedded with a small amount of estrogen. It's easily inserted into the vagina every three months. Body warmth helps the medical silicon slowly release the estrogen into the surrounding tissue. Women can insert the Estring themselves, squeezing it so it resembles a thin figure 8. When inserted properly, women don't feel it. If they do feel it, it's simple enough to use a finger and push it higher up in the vaginal canal. Removal is easy by simply crooking a finger under the ring and pulling it out. The Estring should be removed and replaced every ninety days.

- **VAGIFEM.** These are small tablets of estrogen that are inserted with a disposable applicator directly into the vagina. The tablets adhere to the walls and release the estrogen directly into the vaginal mucosa. Women start by using Vagifem every other day for two weeks, then it's recommended to use Vagifem two times each week. Many women prefer Vagifem because it's convenient, there's less discharge, and it dissolves within hours, so you and your partner don't feel it.

Nurse Barb's Vaginal Comfort Tips

- **INCREASE YOUR BENEFICIAL BACTERIA**—An easy and fast way to help your vagina maintain lots of one type of healthy lactobacilli is to start eating more yogurt with active cultures or take a probiotic with lactobacilli in it.

- **FAST TRACK**—To get lactobacilli into the vagina super fast, insert it directly by dipping your finger into some plain, unflavored yogurt, then swirl that finger in your vagina one to two times each week.

- **LIGHT-SPEED LACTOBACILLI**—If the idea of swirling yogurt in your vagina is unappealing, then dissolve a probiotic capsule in 1 to 2 teaspoons of water that's body temperature. Dip your finger into the dissolved probiotic and then insert that into your vagina one to two times each week. There will be millions to billions of lactobacilli in every drop.

Nurse Barb's Super-Soothing Tips for an Irritated Vulva

- Take cool- to cold-water baths one to four times a day.

- Alternate between soaking in baths that contain Aveeno or a do-it-yourself oatmeal bath and baths using Epsom salts. Both oatmeal and salt help sooth the skin.

- Don't use soap; just soak in your special bath.

- After each bath or visit to the bathroom, do not wipe dry, but gently pat the skin.

- Use a hair dryer on a cool setting to dry the skin.

- Avoid wearing underwear and try wearing a loose-fitting pair of pants or a skirt.

- Apply an ice bag covered with a cotton pillowcase to the vulva. This soothes the skin while protecting it from direct contact with ice, which could further burn and irritate sensitive skin.

- Do not wipe after urination or bowel movements; instead, use a small squirt bottle with water to gently cleanse the skin, and then pat dry.

- Apply a thin layer of diaper ointment or a zinc oxide ointment (such as Balmex) before bed and when the skin is dry.

- Avoid petroleum jelly.

- As much as possible avoid wearing any type of pad in your underwear.

- Wear white cotton underwear; synthetic fibers or dyes can be irritating.

- Use alternative remedies for vaginal dryness, such as aloe vera gel or Neosporin (or its generic counterpart). Although not studied specifically for vaginal dryness, these remedies work for some women to help the outside skin feel better. You can safely use either product one to two times a day.

Nurse Barb's Soothing Sex Tips

- If there's pain with entry and things feel too tight, try having an orgasm first, as that will help the vagina be maximally elongated and receptive to stretching.

- If you bear down, like you're having a particularly difficult bowel movement, your vagina will open up a little to a lot more than normal, which makes it easier to insert tampons, fingers, toys, or even a penis.

- If you can drink or eat it, you can use it with sex. That means olive, vegetable, or other cooking oils can be used as a lubricant.

- If sex is too painful, take a vacation from intercourse. Instead, focus on exploring how other practices such as oral sex and lots of massage can be just as pleasurable for both partners.

- For any irritation, use cool or cold water. Hot water makes it worse because it increases the temperature and the blood flow to the area. Cool water decreases inflammation.

- Stretching the vaginal opening should only be done with patience and plenty of time. It helps to use estrogen treatment for at least six weeks before starting. Use a lubricant, olive oil, or other cooking oil to gently massage the vaginal opening to help it stretch.

- If the vaginal opening has become so small that insertion of a finger, toy, or a penis is impossible, do see a healthcare provider for evaluation and a treatment plan.

DON'T WAIT TO SEEK IMPROVEMENT

What I've found with my patients and what research confirms is that it's never too late to improve conditions and help the sleeping estrogen receptors in the vagina flicker back to life. Even a small improvement can greatly improve a woman's quality of life. As soon as you notice any decrease in your own spontaneous lubrication, ask your healthcare provider to evaluate your vagina and vulva for the beginning signs of dryness. Even if you're still having periods and haven't started having hot flashes and night sweats, we know that as perimenopause and menopause approach, tiny decreases in estrogen are affecting the vagina and vulva. Consider using a small amount of estrogen in the vagina to maintain vaginal health. If hormones aren't an option that you're comfortable with, start a routine with Replens and lots of lubricant. Remember that the more stimulation and blood flow to the area from any sexual activity, including masturbation, will keep the blood and juices flowing to the tissues.

At any time, if conditions spiral out of control and you have pain, itching, or burning or are unable to have sex, then by all means see your healthcare practitioner for help. If you're not getting the help and support you need, go to the North American Menopause Society's website—NAMS.org—to find a certified menopause practitioner.

9

Cooling Off
Without Hormones

Some people call them flashes, and some call them flushes. Whatever you call them, they're no fun and a royal pain in the . . . well, you get the idea. It's hard to feel sexy when your underarms are like faucets and you're sweating through your clothes in nanoseconds. We're definitely hot around menopause, but it's not the "I'm turned on" kind of hot, it's the "100 percent humidity, I'm sweaty and sticky and miserable, don't touch me, I want a cold shower" kind of hot.

For women who've never had a hot flash or a night sweat, it's similar to what you'd experience if you were in a pleasant room at the perfect temperature and you suddenly stepped into a sauna or steam room. There's one important difference though: the heat starts from inside your body, then radiates outward to the surface. Women describe hot flashes as an intense feeling of searing heat that comes on abruptly and out of nowhere. It's as if they have a coal-fired furnace in their chest pumping out BTUs faster than the speed of light.

How each woman experiences hot flashes and night sweats in menopause differs widely. Some women find that the heat smolders slowly at their chest or waist level and then rapidly picks up speed as it travels upward to their face and head and brings with it drenched underarms. Often a racing heartbeat accompanies a hot flash, which can lead to more anxiety and another, you guessed it, hot flash. Other women notice that the heat starts at the back of the neck and then circles around to the front as it moves upward toward the forehead, culminating in a sunburn-like redness and tiny beads of sweat pearling on their upper lips. They may feel heat radiating to their arms and chest. I've heard women describe feeling as if their skin is sizzling with heat. Some women sweat profusely with a hot flash and others shiver.

Night sweats are often more bothersome than hot flashes because they derail restful and rejuvenating sleep, leading to intense daytime irritability and difficulty focusing.

This chapter will discuss many of the same issues that were explored in Chapters 4 and 6, and by necessity, some of the information here may be a review of what you've read in those earlier chapters. However, we'll be adding more information about treatment options that don't involve hormones.

In the past, we doled out hormone treatment like candy on Halloween; that is, until research showed that there was no free lunch. While the benefits of hormone treatment were widely touted, the risks weren't well known and rarely discussed. Many menopausal women are interested in feeling better but aren't even remotely interested in using any hormone treatments. One size never fits all. Many women use a combination of herbs, dietary changes, exercise, acupuncture, and prescription medications to reduce their most bothersome symptoms and enhance their vitality, confidence, and sexiness.

I'd like to introduce you to three of my patients who wanted relief for their drenching hot flashes and night sweats and yet weren't at all interested in using hormones. Joy, Alison, and Shauna had different reasons for choosing the options that ultimately worked for them.

JOY'S STORY

Joy threw off the covers for the fourth time that night. The river of sweat on the back of her neck soaked the pillow, making everything clammy. One minute she was sleeping comfortably and the next she felt that she had been plunged into a steam room. Her skin seemed to sizzle as if molten lava had replaced the blood in her veins. She sighed wearily and got up slowly, heading to the bathroom to empty her bladder. She wasn't sure if it was her full bladder that triggered the night sweat or the night sweat that triggered the sensation of a full bladder. She looked at the sport watch she left on the sink. It was 4:30 AM, and really—who cared what caused what? With a new dry nightgown on, she turned the pillow over to the cool side and slid back into bed. Falling asleep again was a fifty-fifty chance at best. Even though she was bone tired from these constant night sweats that interrupted her sleep night after night, sometimes she needed a full hour to doze off again.

In the morning, Joy felt useless unless she had a few sips of lukewarm coffee. She used to love her coffee piping hot, but since that also led to a hot flash, she settled for a much cooler version. It wasn't as appealing, but the caffeine helped her focus and clear the fog in her head. She headed to the shower. Like her coffee, it, too, was lukewarm, with jets of cold water at the end to help ward off more hot flashes.

Joy had an elaborate system for getting ready for work. She had a fan positioned on the bathroom counter, set at full blast, to keep her nice and cool when she stepped out of her cold shower. This gave her a decent chance of putting on a little makeup without it running off her face in a river of sweat. She waited until the last possible moment to get dressed because of the waterfall pouring out of her underarms. And oceans of sweat on her back had ruined more blouses than what you'd see on a clearance rack at Macy's.

At fifty-two years of age, Joy's hot flashes and night sweats had rolled into her life like a tsunami six months previously. She was still having periods every four to six weeks and was completely unprepared. It was as if a switch had been flipped on and suddenly she was walking around in her own personal steam room.

Joy hoped her hot flashes and night sweats would disappear as quickly as they had arrived. She thought that she could wait them out, but they were getting worse, not better. She came in to see me wanting to know what she could do to get her life back.

After I outlined the menu of options available, Joy decided to try a step-by-step approach. First, she started going to a yoga class once a week and used slow, deep breathing as soon as she felt the onset of a hot flash. At the same time, she increased her soy intake by snacking on roasted soy nuts while making dinner. After a month, she called to say that she noticed a slight improvement, but not as much as she had hoped for. That's when she decided to try Remifemin, a black cohosh herbal supplement that has been studied as a remedy for hot flashes. (See Lifestyle Remedies later in this chapter for more about black cohosh.)

After another month, she was somewhat better, but still waking three to four times each night. Next, Joy decided to try using an antidepressant to reset her internal thermostat. Though Joy didn't have any history of depression or anxiety, several of her friends were on various types of anti-depressants without complaining of any problems. I suggested that she begin Pristiq at a low dose, and then after three weeks increase it if she was still having symptoms. I explained that though there was a lot of research that showed that Pristiq was effective, it didn't have FDA approval for use for hot flashes and I'd be prescribing it to her "off label."

"I appreciate that you told me that," she said. "Otherwise when I did my own online research, I might have freaked out a bit. As long as it works and is safe, I want to give it a go." I checked back with Joy after another month, and it was like talking to a whole new person. "I'm finally sleeping!" she exclaimed. "I'm only having one to two night sweats a week, not four every night, and because they're mild it's so much easier to fall back to sleep. The best part is my hot flashes have virtually disappeared. I might have one a week now, instead of three every hour. I feel so much more energetic and a lot less crabby. I'm happy to have something that works without worrying about the issues with hormones."

ALISON'S STORY

Alison sat in bumper-to-bumper traffic fuming. She hated her morning commute and was trying to reach for her latest book on tape, feeling angry with all the other drivers crowding around her. Then she felt a sudden wave of intense, searing heat that began around her stomach and traveled up her chest, her neck, and finally burst out the top of her head. She cranked up the air conditioning thinking it would pass, when another wave of heat ignited in the pit of her stomach, culminating in a layer of sweat pouring down her back and soaking her clothes.

Alison knew that stress could trigger a hot flash, but this was ridiculous. She could barely think about a work project or anything even remotely *stressful when within seconds she'd feel her skin vibrating with heat and her heart beating rapidly.*

Prior to her transformation into a pizza oven, she had never been conscious of her heartbeat, yet now a hot flash brought with it a racing heart and a low roaring sound in her ears. Anything could trigger a hot flash, from mild stress to sitting in a hot car. She'd also noticed that anytime she drank red wine she paid for the pleasure with a sopping neck and red face.

At fifty-two, Alison's periods arrived sporadically. She only had had three in the last year. With two to seven night sweats each night and clusters of hot flashes, she felt like she was going crazy and that her daily life was out of control. She was ready for relief when she came in to see me.

Alison worked as a mammography technician. Her patients, especially the ones battling breast cancer, shared their strategies for coping with hot flashes. She knew enough from the women who had chemotherapy-induced symptoms to avoid all the hot flash triggers. Alison was adamant; there was no way she'd even consider using hormones. She wanted to try every other option first. She then listed all the things she already did to eliminate hot flash triggers that weren't working. She took cold showers, stuffed cool packs into her pillows, and had her husband start the car and blast the air conditioner for her before she jumped in. She was also doing regular yoga breathing and had an appointment to see an acupuncturist who specialized in women's issues. She was hopeful that a personalized mix of herbs would be more effective than the black cohosh she had tried previously, which had little effect.

Alison came back in after three months. The acupuncturist was helping her get her qi ("chi") in alignment. In the meantime, her hot flashes had reduced by about 25 percent, which was a good start, but she still wanted more relief. I suggested that she try S-Equol, a new supplement made from a metabolite of the soy isoflavone daidzein. Research has shown that many women have marked improvement in their hot flashes and muscle aches after taking S-Equol. I tried it myself after reviewing the safety data and found that it worked well for me with no side effects.

After two months taking S-Equol, Alison felt like herself again. She still had a few hot flashes each week, but they were more manageable. She couldn't remember the last time she felt her heart racing or had roaring in her ears.

SHAUNA'S STORY

My neighbor Shauna's experience with menopause began so suddenly, it was like a switch had been flipped when she had surgery to remove her ovaries after her breast cancer went into remission. On the advice of her oncologist, Shauna had been tested for the presence of the breast cancer genetic mutations BRCA1 and BRCA2, which are associated with a high risk of breast cancer occurrence. Because she tested positive for one of the BRCA genetic mutations, she was at high risk for not only a recurrence of breast cancer, but for ovarian cancer as well. Then, because she had her ovaries removed—thus removing her body's source of estrogen—she experienced menopause in the blink of an eye. By the time she came home from the hospital, she was living in a perpetual steam room. Shauna wasn't just hot, she was boiling over. She thought that dealing with her breast cancer and the radiation had been a challenge, but this was putting her over the edge. She knew that her oncologist would have a heart attack if she asked for hormones, and she didn't want to do anything that would lead to another cancer, but she was desperate.

Shauna was barely sleeping and had resorted to using sleeping pills, but those made her groggy in the mornings. She was beyond tired and was becoming increasingly irritable. She felt like she was constantly using yoga breathing and yet nothing she did seemed to help. Shauna took at least two cool showers each day and stowed a tiny battery-operated fan in her purse. She didn't have air conditioning in her house but loved to stand in front of the open fridge door when things got particularly bad. It was a nightmare, and there were no signs that she'd wake up cooler and more comfortable anytime soon.

Shauna searched online for answers but was confused by all the various claims and conflicting opinions. I had no idea that she was suffering until I dropped off some lasagna for the family and shared some iced tea with her. I was surprised that none of her doctors had offered her any nonhormonal options for the relief of her hot flashes. "They told me that it would pass," she explained. "I'm just trying to hang on as best I can."

I just shook my head and then we launched into a discussion of all the various nonhormonal remedies available to her that weren't associated with any risk of breast cancer. She had already tried soy and was intrigued by the idea of using gabapentin, a medication that's been used for a variety of things from reducing pain to preventing seizures. Though it doesn't have FDA approval to reduce hot flashes and night sweats, many women with breast cancer have found relief, especially at night. Shauna contacted her oncologist who recommended one nighttime dose, since one of the side effects of gabapentin is drowsiness. Within weeks, Shauna was sleeping through most nights, which helped her manage the hot flashes that occurred throughout the day.

THE NITTY-GRITTY ON COOLING OFF WITHOUT HORMONES

As you may recall from my earlier discussion, a hot flash is actually the body's mixed-up attempt at cooling off. With declining estrogen levels, the brain's thermostat and temperature regulation system go a bit haywire. Prior to menopause, drinking a cup of hot coffee or taking a hot shower wouldn't cause the brain to trigger a cooling-off cascade of events, but that's what happens in menopause. Now even tiny changes in temperature, as little as 0.5 degrees can start the sweats. Prior to menopause, a woman's body can tolerate a few degrees of temperature change or stressful thoughts without sweating.

When the brain wants the body to cool off quick, it initiates a cooling-off cascade; blood vessels near the surface of the skin quickly dilate to cool off the circulating blood, sweat glands become activated to help dissipate the heat, and often the heart will beat more rapidly. It all adds up to a flush or flash of intense heat and possibly sweating, shivering, and a racing heart. Researchers believe that hot flashes begin when neurotransmitters, such as norepinephrine and serotonin are released after a triggering event.

A Menu of Nonhormonal Treatment Options

My approach with all of my patients who have hot flashes and night sweats is to provide them with a menu of options that range from the simple prevention of hot flash triggers to incorporating natural herbs, supplements, and foods into their diet, and includes a list of prescription medications and hormones. However, this chapter focuses on only the nonhormonal remedies. See the next chapter for my menu of hormonal options.

* *

Rapid Menopause from Surgery or Breast Cancer Treatment

For women who have a sudden loss of hormones when the ovaries are surgically removed, or from breast cancer treatment, the intensity and frequency of hot flashes and night sweats usually arrive like a bullet train. It's typically a fast and furious introduction to menopause and can be quite overwhelming. It's important to help these women be aware that there are options available that can help, and that they need to start them as soon as possible.

* *

You may wonder why some women can successfully treat their hot flashes with obscure and crazy remedies and yet you can't find any credible evidence that they work. The truth is, every study on hot flash and night sweat remedies finds one consistent result; there's a tremendous placebo effect with virtually every remedy studied. (The placebo effect is a beneficial effect that cannot be attributed to the ingredient itself, but rather to a person's belief that the treatment is effective.) The placebo effect in most studies for menopause remedies ranges from 30 to 50 percent. That means that we could test the effect of drinking tap water on hot flashes, and you'd probably find that about 30 percent of women saw a reduction in their hot flashes compared to women who drank filtered water.

As I describe treatment options here, I only include those that have been shown to be more effective than placebo treatments. However, if you find that doing cartwheels works or that some obscure herb in your cup of tea is beneficial without any negative side effects, then by all means use it.

Nurse Barb's Nonhormonal Remedy Menu

Prevention

• Recognizing and avoiding hot flash triggers

Lifestyle remedies

• Deep breathing

• Acupuncture

Foods and Herbs

• Black Cohosh

• Soy

• S-Equol

• Flaxseed

Medications available by prescription

• Antidepressants—Paroxetine (Brisdelle) has been approved by the FDA to treat hot flashes and night sweats in menopause

• Gabapentin

Ice Cold Tips

• Staying cool with whatever's on hand

Recognizing and Avoiding Triggers

In menopause, I'm all about prevention, and this applies to every strategy I recommend when advising women how to deal with their hot flashes and night sweats. It's better to stay cool and avoid the flash than have to deal with the sweat pouring out. Hot flashes and night sweats can be triggered by just about anything from a random thought to trying on a sweater. Though each woman will have her own personal list of triggers for hot flashes, there are a few that are common for all of us. They include the following:

- A hot shower

- Any increase in temperature

- Becoming overheated

- Being in the hot sun

- Drinking a warm or hot beverage

- Drinking alcohol

- Drinking caffeinated beverages

- Eating spicy foods

- Sex

- Sitting in a hot car

- Smoking

- Standing next to a heater or any heat source

- Stress, worry, anxiety

- Using a hair dryer

- Wearing more than a thin layer of clothing

Avoiding these triggers will reduce your hot flashes and just may be the right recipe for handling them with ease. See the end of the chapter for Nurse Barb's Keeping Cool Tips—guaranteed to turn down the heat for more comfortable days and nights.

Lifestyle Remedies

Many of the nonhormonal remedies listed below have been used by women with breast cancer who weren't able to use estrogen. After listening to women's stories about what worked for them, researchers started digging deeper, looking for evidence to back up the claims. I feel a personal debt of gratitude to the thousands of breast cancer survivors and other women who participated in these studies so that we could all benefit from the findings.

- **TAKE A DEEP BREATH**—For both prevention and treatment, numerous studies found that the regular practice of slow, deep breathing, similar to what is done with yoga, will decrease hot flashes. It's also been shown that if a woman slows down her breathing to approximately six deep breaths per minute as soon as she feels a hot flash starting, then the intensity and duration will be decreased. We're not sure exactly how this works; however, it's likely that slow, deep breathing decreases the output of stress hormones and neurotransmitters that trigger and worsen hot flashes. By making a regular practice of deep breathing throughout the day, women can also reduce the number and severity of hot flashes and night sweats.

- **ACUPUNCTURE**—Very well-controlled research has documented that acupuncture works to decrease the number, frequency, and intensity of hot flashes and night sweats by adjusting the *qi* ("chi"), which is defined as the natural or essential life force. I've seen an acupuncturist myself, and I've recommended acupuncture to my menopausal patients because there are studies that show benefit and many women have reported back to me that they feel better. Though acupuncture may not completely eliminate hot flashes and night sweats, many women find they're decreased to a level that's much easier to cope with.

- **VITAMIN E**—There's controversy about whether vitamin E is a reliable remedy for menopausal symptoms. There have been studies that demonstrate only a slight benefit with vitamin E at doses that range from 400 to 800 IU per day. Other studies show no benefit over a placebo. Because vitamin E is stored in our fat, it's best to check with your healthcare provider or pharmacist about whether it's a safe option for you. Vitamin E may interact with aspirin, nonsteroidal anti-inflammatory medications such as Advil, Aleve, or Motrin, and the anticoagulant Coumadin (warfarin).

- **BLACK COHOSH**—Numerous studies have shown that the herb black cohosh is a more effective treatment for hot flashes than placebo, and yet many other studies don't show a benefit. I've seen that some my patients respond immediately and have a significant reduction in symptoms, while others will not, despite increasing the dose or the amount of time they use it. It's puzzling, and yet my theory is that some women probably have a receptor for some yet undiscovered nutrient in black cohosh, making them more likely to respond. If you decide to try black cohosh, my recommendation is to use Remifemin, which has very high manufacturing standards, guaranteeing a consistent dose in each tablet.

  There are two drugs that can cause major drug interactions with black cohosh: Antabuse (disulfiram), which is a medication used to treat alcoholism, and Arava (lefunomide), a medication used to treat rheumatoid arthritis.

- **SOY**—Soybeans are an amazing food. They are the only plant source of complete protein with all nine essential amino acids. They also are a great source of isoflavones, which are a class of phytoestrogens, otherwise known as plant-based estrogens. The active ingredients are genistein and daidzen, which have been shown to decrease hot flashes and night sweats in numerous studies. It's been known for years that women in Asian countries who have a high lifetime intake of soy products have fewer hot flashes and night sweats. As more women in the West looked East for nonhormonal remedies for their menopausal symptoms, the use of soy increased. The latest Dietary Guidelines for Americans from the U.S. Department of Agriculture (USDA) and Department of Health and Human Services (HHS) recommend incorporating soy protein as an alternative to meat into our daily diet to decrease calories and fat. Having at least one daily serving of soy has been recommended by the Food and Drug Administration (FDA) to help decrease total and LDL ("bad") cholesterol.

  For hot flashes and night sweats, I recommend that women add one to two servings of whole soy in the form of soymilk, edamame, tofu, roasted soy nuts, or other soy food into their daily diet. Many patients have seen a significant reduction in symptoms in a few weeks.

There have been some suggestions in the research that women who haven't had soy as children and then begin to eat three or more servings a day in menopause may have an increased risk of breast cancer, because of the estrogen-like effects in the isoflavones that has been seen in studies with animals. To date, the research on soy doesn't show any increased risk of breast cancer, even in women who've had breast cancer and are on Tamoxifen or aromatase inhibitors.

Soy is not recommended for people who are on MAO inhibitors (such as Marplan or Nardil) or Coumadin (warfarin) as soy can interfere with the actions of those medications.

• **S-EQUOL**—When we consume certain types of soy, our bodies convert it to a metabolite known as S-equol, which fights off hot flashes and night sweats. The trouble is, only 20 to 30 percent of Caucasian women have the ability to metabolize soy into S-equol. That might explain why some women find relief from soy and others don't. In fact, women who have the ability to convert soy into S-equol have fewer hot flashes.

S-equol and soy do not carry any increased risks of blood clots, heart disease, or breast cancer, making them a safe alternative to battling hot flashes and night sweats. Women who aren't able to produce S-equol on their own can take an S-equol supplement to help reduce their symptoms.

I've tried this myself and found that it worked very well to reduce my own hot flashes and debilitating night sweats. It took about four weeks for me to see the benefit. Because it's hormone free, I recommend that my patients try it as an alternative to other treatments. Just as people on MAO inhibitors and Coumadin should avoid soy, I recommend the same for S-equol.

• **FLAXSEED**—This legume is an incredible multitasking nutrient. It's not only loaded with omega-3 fatty acids in the form of alpha-linolenic acid, it is also a lignan, which like soy is another phytoestrogen or plant source of estrogen.

Research has shown that consuming ground flaxseed can decrease hot flashes and night sweats as well as help lower cholesterol. Flaxseed has a laxative-like effect and is very effective in stimulating the intestines, so it's a good idea to start with a small amount and gradually increase what you take in, to prevent a lot of trips to the bathroom.

The benefit of flaxseed is that there is no increased risk of breast cancer or blood clots. However, there are many possible drug interactions, so it's best to check with your pharmacist or healthcare provider before starting it. Flaxseed can interact with aspirin, blood-thinning medications such as Coumadin (warfarin), Heparin, Lovenox, Plavix, nonsteroidal anti-inflammatory medications such as Advil and Motrin, drugs that treat diabetes, and many other medications.

Prescription Medications

Many women start by incorporating the lifestyle remedies that are listed above to reduce hot flashes and night sweats. For some women, it's enough to add herbs or soy to their diet to relieve symptoms. Many others, however, are still looking for other effective options that do not involve hormones.

- **ANTIDEPRESSANTS**—Women with breast cancer who were taking antidepressants for depression and anxiety found a surprising improvement in their hot flashes. This sparked more study with more promising results. There are several types of antidepressant medications that have been shown in numerous well-controlled studies to decrease hot flashes and night sweats, including the selective serotonin reuptake inhibitors (SSRIs) and the selective serotonin and norepinephrine reuptake inhibitors (SNRIs). These medications help us retain more serotonin and/or more norepinephrine, which are neurotransmitters. These influence our body's own temperature regulation and thermostat.

  We believe that both SSRIs and SNRIs widen the thermoneutral zone (TNZ) and help women reset their personal thermostat (see Chapter 6). Our body's natural thermostat is located in the area of the brain that is also influenced by the neurotransmitters serotonin and norepinephrine. By keeping serotonin and norepinephrine around longer and inhibiting their rapid clearance, women in menopause can reset their thermostats and decrease their hot flashes. Studies demonstrated that both of these types of antidepressants are significantly better than a placebo in reducing both the frequency and severity of hot flashes and night sweats as well as improving quality of life and sleep.

Recently, the Food and Drug Administration (FDA) approved the first nonhormonal medication—the antidepressant paroxetine (Brisdelle)—as a treatment for hot flashes and night sweats in menopause. This is the only antidepressant that's been approved for this indication.

To treat menopausal symptoms, the dosages that are typically used in paroxetine and other antidepressants are lower than what is used to treat depression. To stave off the most common side effect, nausea and stomach upset, I recommend that my patients start at a low dose and then gradually work up to a level of medication that is safe and decreases their symptoms. The nausea and stomach upset typically resolve after two to three weeks.

Probably the most important benefit of using a SSRI or SNRI antidepressant is that using them does not increase the risk of breast cancer, blood clots, or any other potentially serious side effects. They are a safe alternative to estrogen therapy, which though more effective, also carries some significant risks. Women who use antidepressants should discuss possible drug interactions with their healthcare provider or pharmacist.

Researchers have studied the question of whether SSRI antidepressant use is associated with an increased risk of suicide—a topic that also has been in the press. A review of the data, however, doesn't show that this is a risk factor in adults. There is some cause for concern for increased suicide risk among teens and children taking these medications, and research studies about this are ongoing.

Many women shy away from the option of taking antidepressants because of the perceived stigma attached to using these medications and the conscious or unconscious shame that we are somehow "less than" if we need to use a medication that's associated with emotional health to help our symptoms. It can be more troubling because of the perception that using an antidepressant for hot flashes means that we are actually crazy. This is an unfortunate way to think about using a medication that works because you don't have to be crazy, depressed, or anxious to have hot flashes and night sweats, and more important, these medications work. Improved sleep and increased energy are two other benefits that many women find when using an antidepressant. There have also been some case reports of improved sex drive.

The fact is that during menopause, our ride on the hormonal roller coaster affects the neurotransmitters in our brains, leading to many bothersome symptoms, including depression. Some of my patients have become more aware of a lingering depression that they've coped with for years prior to menopause, but that became less manageable as hormonal changes at midlife affected their sleep and mood. There are many women who are not depressed and use antidepressants to help them sleep and control hot flashes and night sweats. There are also many women who have depression, are treated with antidepressants, and have the side benefit of obtaining relief from menopausal symptoms. It's important to discuss any change in mood or depressed feelings with your healthcare provider.

For women who are not interested in a hormonal option for treating hot flashes and night sweats, using an antidepressant may be a good alternative. They work simply by adjusting the way our body utilizes the neurotransmitters that affect the thermoneutral zone (TNZ) *and* our mood. I understand the hesitation in using these medications; however, in my experience there are many benefits and few risks.

FDA-Approved for Menopause

SSRIs (selective serotonin reuptake inhibitors): Brisdelle (paroxetine)

Non-FDA-Approved and Used Off-Label

SSRIs (selective serotonin reuptake inhibitors): Lexapro (escitalopram), Prozac (fluoxetine), Zoloft (sertraline)

SNRIs (selective serotonin and norepinephrine reuptake inhibitors): Effexor XR (venlafaxine), Pristiq (desvenlafaxine), Cymbalta (duloxetine)

Possible drug interactions:

Imitrex, Theophylline, Xanax, Codeine, Coumadin, Tegretol (carbemazepine), Mellaril (thioridazine), Beta blockers (medications for high blood pressure or heart disease)

- **GABAPENTIN**—Many women with breast cancer and those on chemo-therapy have found relief from their hot flashes and night sweats by using gabapentin, also known under its brand name Neurontin. We think it works by widening the TNZ. Studies have shown that gabapentin can reduce hot flashes and night sweats as much as 70 percent, and it allows women to sleep better at night. Many of the studies that have been done also showed a very high placebo effect, which is probably why the FDA has not approved gabapentin as a remedy for hot flashes and night sweats. One of gabapentin's side effects is that it causes drowsiness—which is a great side effect and possible solution for women with night sweats.

  Drugs that interact with gabapentin include aspirin and Tylenol (acetaminophen). Women with kidney disease need to check with their healthcare provider about whether gabapentin is safe to use.

What Are "Off-Label" Prescriptions?

When a medication is approved by the U.S. Food and Drug Administration (FDA), it's generally approved for certain indications, symptoms, illnesses, or conditions. The FDA, which is around to protect us from false claims about drugs, is very careful to only approve medication for an indication when there is sufficient evidence that it works, which is considered "on-label use."

Pharmaceutical companies are prohibited from saying that the medication works for other indications, which are "off-label" until the FDA is satisfied that the data supports those other claims. In the meantime though, research reported in journals, conferences, and symposia supports the "off-label" use. So even though a drug may be approved by the FDA and be in the drugstore, the reason or indication for its use may be considered "off-label."

Nevertheless, many healthcare providers prescribe many medications for off-label indications, including hot flashes and night sweats.

Nurse Barb's Keeping Cool Tips

- **TURNING OFF THE SWEAT**—If your deodorant isn't up to the challenge of menopause, look for a strong antiperspirant with the active ingredient aluminum zirconium tetrachlorohydrex gly. You don't need to be able to pronounce it to know that it works.

- **AVOID DRINKING HOT BEVERAGES**—Become a fan of iced coffee or cold tea in the morning if you need the jolt of caffeine. If you must have hot coffee, you can sometimes avoid a hot flash by having a big gulp of cold water after your first few sips of hot liquid.

- **AVOID ALCOHOL, ESPECIALLY IN THE EVENING**—Pay attention to what types of alcohol cause your hot flashes. Many women find that one type of alcohol triggers a hot flash and/or a headache, but others are less bothersome. Many of my friends and patients can't drink red wine, but tolerate champagne and vodka. Others find that white wine is their new favorite happy-hour drink.

- **AVOID DEHYDRATION**—This occurs with exercise, alcohol, and caffeine. Bring along plenty of water whenever you exercise. If you're having any alcohol, have two full glasses of water for every cocktail or beer you enjoy. Alcohol in the evening may not lead to immediate hot flashes but will instead make you pay the price with night sweats later on. Even though it means more trips to the bathroom, stay hydrated.

- **AVOID LARGE EVENING MEALS**—Maybe it's the signal from a distended stomach that triggers hot flashes or just the added work of digestion, but a heavy meal means hot flashes and night sweats for dessert. If you're like most women dealing with some menopausal weight gain, smaller portions are an essential lifestyle change anyway.

- **AVOID SPICY FOOD**—If you like your food piping hot or spicy hot, you may have to look for other ways to tantalize your taste buds. Use other spices for flavor that doesn't make you sweat, or if you absolutely must have the cayenne pepper or hot sauce, have some cold beer, cold milk, or yogurt as a chaser to turn down the heat.

- **COLD SHOWERS**—Start your shower off warm, so that you don't get chilled, and then gradually lower the temperature. Then, if you can tolerate it, rinse in the coldest water you can stand and soak your head and neck in cold water before stepping out of the shower.

- **INVEST IN GOOD QUALITY SHEETS**—To help stay cool while sleeping and avoid night sweats, skip the flannel nightgown and wear the most lightweight clothes possible. High-thread-count sheets will be cooler than the ones with a lower thread count. Shop the sales.

- **CHILLED CUCUMBERS**—Eating cold and chilled fruits and vegetables cools you off in two important ways. First, the natural juiciness keeps you hydrated, and second, chilled foods cool from the inside out. Try chilled gazpacho, Italian ices, and cold lemonade. Don't you feel cooler already? You can also lie down and place cool cucumber slices over your eyes and practice deep breathing—guaranteed to bring calm, cool relief.

- **HAIR AND MAKEUP**—Be sure to have a cold fan running in the bathroom to keep you cool while you towel off, moisturize, dry your hair, and put on your makeup. Let your hair air dry as much as possible before getting out the hairdryer, and use styling products and rollers to get things started if possible. I have patients who keep ice cubes in a bowl to rub on their wrists to cool off when getting ready in the morning. Others plunge their wrists under cold running water for a quick cool off.

- **ARCTIC ADJUSTMENTS TO YOUR THERMOSTAT**—Turn down the ambient heat in your home, office, and car whenever possible. Everyone else around you can wear a sweater.

- **COLD PACKS**—You can slip a cool pack under your pillowcase. There are cooling pillows available online, too. Chilling a pillowcase in the freezer and sleeping on a nice cold pillow can help you start the night off a few degrees cooler. Look for other cooling products that you can wear under your clothes or keep in your car or office for quick cooling.

- **SEEK OUT THE SHADE**—Wear a hat, look for shade, and if you know you're going to be in a place where there's hot sun, bring a light-colored umbrella, personal fan, lots of extra water, and whatever else you need to be comfortable, including personal cold packs.

- **DRESS LIKE AN ONION AND PEEL OFF THE LAYERS**—This seems like a no-brainer, but many times we forget that a thin sleeveless shell or tank can be layered with a blouse and then a jacket so that we can peel off the layers as needed.

- **LOOK AT THE LABELS**—There are many new fabrics that wick moisture away from the body and are lightweight enough to prevent getting over-heated. Avoid silk, cashmere, and wool, and trend toward light cottons and thin jersey materials that are looser, which helps air circulate. Avoid tights if possible and consider skirts, not slacks.

- **DON'T SMOKE AND AVOID SECONDHAND SMOKE**—Smoking triggers hot flashes and so does being around secondhand smoke. Fresh air, a fan, and open windows are the best remedy.

●   ●   ●   ●   ●   ●   ●   ●   ●   ●   ●   ●   ●   ●   ●   ●

FEEL BETTER NATURALLY

Hot flashes and night sweats are no fun. They can wreak havoc on our days and nights for years and affect quality of life. Women can feel hot and sexy again as soon as they're not feeling hot and sweaty. The good news is that these symptoms will eventually diminish and decrease, but they often hit us just when we're hitting our stride personally and professionally. Many women don't have the luxury of waiting for these bothersome symptoms to subside but are looking for natural, nonhormonal, and safe ways to manage them. There are a variety of treatment options available, from yoga, breathing, and acupuncture to S-Equol, gabapentin, and antidepressants.

Many women start with a step-by-step approach, beginning by avoiding triggers and breathing deeply, perhaps adding in soy or black cohosh for a few months. Others will have suffered for months and are ready for a prescription medication that helps symptoms and helps them get the restful sleep they need. No matter what you choose to do, find the remedy or combination of treatments that work with your lifestyle. Getting some sleep, regaining energy, and feeling your best is the greatest gift you can give yourself.

10

Staying Cool with Hormonal Options

$\mathcal{T}$hough many women are able to glide through menopause without any major upheavals, there are others who have an experience more akin to what passengers on the *Titanic* must have felt; their world suddenly turned upside down. Very severe hot flashes and night sweats arrive suddenly and leave them worn out, tired, dripping in sweat, and miserable for years. For women with severe symptoms, finding the right treatment option feels like being rescued by a lifeboat; they literally get their lives back.

It's as if they woke up one day feeling like a completely different person. They can't sleep, are extremely irritable, and have trouble concentrating. Also included at no additional charge: A personal internal sauna set at six thousand degrees that switches on and off without warning, especially when it's least convenient. It's impossible to feel hot and sexy when you're hot and clammy, have had no sleep, and are so irritable that people around you know to keep their distance.

During menopause, there are no guarantees of having a decent day or a restful night. Women don't know if they'll toss and turn in a sweat-soaked nightgown for two hours and finally drift off to sleep at 4 AM or manage to eke out five to six hours of uninterrupted sleep on any given night. They wonder if their foundation will stay put or run off down their neck with the first or thirteenth hot flash of the day. They're also not completely sure if their irritability is as obvious to their family and friends as it is to them. And yet, there are some experiences that are predictable. For example, they'll probably sweat through at least one blouse each week. They can pretty much guarantee that a hot flash will erupt like a lava flow anytime they drink a cup of hot coffee or tea. In addition, any stressful situation from a parent-teacher meeting to a major presentation is likely to bring on a racing heart, beads of sweat pearling on a reddened forehead, and a slight feeling of panic. It's no surprise that women dealing with these types of tumultuous upheavals will do just about anything, short of standing on their heads in the middle of traffic, to relieve their symptoms and reclaim some control over their lives.

With mild symptoms, women can shrug off the occasional disruption of a hot flash or the interrupted sleep from the rare night sweat and not seek treatment options. However, for women with severe symptoms, whose lives are in upheaval, relief cannot come fast enough. These women want their lives back right now! They are looking for the most effective options for relief of their hormonal roller-coaster ride of symptoms. The good news is that we have a very effective treatment for hot flashes and night sweats: estrogen.

Hold on, though—there is some bad news. Unfortunately, using estrogen is a package deal that includes some rare but serious risks. With hormonal treatments, there's no free lunch, because while using estrogen to relieve menopausal symptoms is very effective, there are possible worrisome side effects. There's been a pendulum of advice on hormonal treatments over the last ten to twelve years. If it seems as if the prevailing winds of thought on hormones change every six months, it's because they **DO.** If the experts can't agree on whether hormones are safe, then how can we expect women, who are busy with their own lives, to be able to sift through all of the conflicting information and opinions and make informed choices? I think it's a lot to ask, and that's where I can help.

The two biggest problems that my patients encounter are these: Number one, there is no one clear-cut choice that works for every single woman that is completely risk free. Second, while there are lots of studies on hormones, there aren't any side-by-side comparisons of various women at various ages using various hormone preparations, which makes it impossible to put all of the information into context for each unique and individual woman. This chapter offers an overview of hormonal options. For a deeper dive into the nitty-gritty of the differences in various hormonal options, including bioidentical and compounded hormones, see Chapter 11 and the appendix.

When considering whether to use hormones to treat menopausal symptoms such as hot flashes, night sweats, shivering, muscle aches, or others, it helps to hear how other women made their decisions. Meet Susan, Jen, and Lena, who all had to weigh the risks and benefits of using a prescription hormonal treatment.

SUSAN'S STORY

Susan woke up sopping wet for the third time that night and trudged to the bathroom. Her thin nightgown was damp and clinging to her body. She was tempted to jump into an ice-cold shower but quickly dismissed the idea as being impractical. Besides, she reasoned, then she'd fully wake up and could kiss good-bye any chance of getting back to sleep that night. She'd have to settle for running cold water over her wrist and trying to find yet another fresh nightgown without turning on the light.

Susan had tried increasing her soy intake and was now taking vitamin E to try to ease her hot flashes. She had been going to an acupuncturist for the last four months. Twice daily, she dutifully swallowed the special Chinese herb mixture that tasted awful, but was supposed to help restore her qi ("chi") or essential life force. Though she had a few less hot flashes and night sweats, she was still miserably hot and not getting the relief she had hoped for. The only time she felt comfortable was when she opened up her fridge and stood in front of it cooling off. Otherwise, she felt as if she were living at the equator, with sizzling skin and an internal thermostat permanently set at 105 degrees, except when she had an occasional burst of heat that boiled over into the 120-degree zone.

When it came to sex (though she was up all night), she had zero interest, and what was worse for her was that she didn't care. Her libido had disappeared just as suddenly as the hot flashes arrived. Susan was desper-

ate when she came in for an appointment. "I'm moving to Alaska," she announced as she sat down. "The only time that I've felt like myself was on a cruise to Alaska. Sure, the wildlife was awesome, but the 55-degree days and the 40-degree nights were what sold me. I was outside in a T-shirt day and night and never felt better."

After reviewing the risks and benefits of using various treatment options, Susan was quite sure she didn't want to have hot flashes but was worried about the risks of using hormones. As we discussed the research, Susan became more reassured that the likelihood of serious side effects from hormone treatment was much lower for younger, healthier women than what had been seen in older women with high blood pressure and those who smoked. "I need to function," she said. Once she understood that the vast majority of younger women do well on hormones with far fewer risks, it was easier for her to make a decision about treatment options.

We also discussed the current recommendations—to use the lowest effective dose for the shortest duration of time necessary. She opted to use a transdermal estrogen patch, which she would place on her abdomen and change twice each week. I recommended an FDA-approved bioidentical patch that comes in various strengths. Because she had a uterus, she would also need to use progesterone to balance the possible side effects of the estrogen on the uterine lining. I prescribed Prometrium, a micronized progesterone for her to take every night. This medication has the added benefit of causing mild drowsiness, which would also help her sleep through any feelings of warmth. Taking it every night would also reduce the likelihood of bleeding, which was appealing to her.

When I called Susan two weeks later, she was getting more sleep than she had in months, her hot flashes had virtually disappeared, and her energy was returning, presumably from catching up on sleep. When she came in after six months, she said that she had also found her long-lost sex drive. This was a happy bonus from starting hormones that she hadn't expected. "I'm not sure if we're having more sex because I'm finally able to sleep, or because I'm not scaring him off with my crazy moods, but who cares. Now I don't have to move to Alaska."

JEN'S STORY

Jen gritted her teeth and tried to breathe slowly. She was on the verge of saying something unkind, which would make everything worse. Her super-efficient assistant had just brought her the wrong file. In her rational mind, Jen knew that it wasn't the end of the world, and yet she wanted to lash out and vent some of her building frustration.

Another five deep breaths and her anger cooled enough to prevent an eruption. Widely regarded as the type of attorney who was patient and easy to work with, lately she had been so irritable that the new paralegals were afraid of her. She wondered if it was the lack of sleep from the perpetual night sweats. The hot flashes that passed through her body a few times an hour weren't helping. "I wonder if I'm in a science fiction movie where my body has been switched with someone else's?" she mused. "Someone I don't recognize, someone who's hot, sweaty, and crabby."

Jen ticked off how bedtimes now meant a nightmare of sleepless nights, the fallout from her irritability, and the surprise of repeated hot flashes that came on like tornados a few times an hour. "I can't function like this," she explained. "I want to know what's going on and more impor-tant, I want my life back."

Jen wasn't sure if she was in menopause. She wondered if her thyroid gland was out of whack, if she was going crazy, or if she had picked up some kind of virus. As a lawyer she was used to doing a lot of research, but in this case, she was too tired and too overwhelmed with her work to look into this on her own. She wanted answers and solutions. With a few years of irregular periods, some increasing vaginal dryness, and normal thy-roid levels it was clear that Jen was in the throes of menopause.

"I didn't want to believe that I was old enough to be menopausal. I just don't see myself as someone at midlife," Jen explained. "I'm not at all inter-ested in suffering through these symptoms for months or years. I want them gone now and I'll deal with any side effects." She was surprised that the risks of using hormones weren't as prevalent as she had assumed. I explained it this way. . . .

According to studies, women who use hormones have a slightly increased risk of developing breast cancer, heart disease, blood clots, and stroke. It's estimated that:

- For every 100 women who **Do Not** take hormones, approximately 2 will develop each of these serious conditions in a year.

- For every 100 women who **Do** take hormones, approximately 3 will develop each of these serious conditions in a year.

- That means that for women who take hormones, 1 extra woman per 100 will develop breast cancer, stroke, heart disease, or blood clots.

Jen decided that the risks of using estrogen were remote enough that she'd trade that worry for a decent night's sleep. She began a very low-dose estrogen gel that she applied to her thigh every morning. Because she had her uterus, she also needed to balance the estrogen gel with progesterone to help decrease the risk of developing endometrial cancer in her uterus. Prometrium was a good option, as it would also help her sleep.

Within days, Jen was sleeping six to seven hours each night and only rarely got up to use the bathroom. Initially, she wondered if she was still having night sweats and just sleeping through them, but then she noticed that her skin wasn't clammy in the morning and the damp nightgowns from the past were now completely dry. Within weeks, Jen's mood improved dramatically as her hot flashes disappeared. She hadn't lost her temper at work, and her assistant wasn't shrinking away when Jen approached her with a request. "Amazing what a little sleep will do for a person," she quipped. When I saw her next at her annual physical, Jen decided to stay on her hormone gel. She felt relieved that she was able to find relief that worked without experiencing any serious side effects.

LENA'S STORY

Lena walked out of the coffee shop with her secret weapon, a caramel latte to boost her energy for her afternoon series of carpool treks. Her three kids in middle and high school had overlapping sports and after-school activities, which meant that she was juggling schedules, meals, snacks, smelly uniforms, and a minivan full of other kids. She had a color-coded calendar that kept her on track and organized. She'd long ago learned to put dinner in the crockpot in the morning before heading off to *her part-time job. She knew from years of experience that three kids meant that there was always a last minute change in plans, which meant shuffling the schedule, being flexible, and carrying around extra socks, water bottles, and ice packs that inevitably solved someone's crisis.*

Lena was used to rolling with whatever came her way and not complaining. The trouble was that her little caffeine jolt at 3 PM meant hot flashes and the need to peel off layers of clothes while cranking up the AC and speeding off to the next field. She cringed when she realized that she should have ordered this latte iced.

She hadn't used an epidural for her three deliveries and didn't like to take any medication unless she was dying. Lena wasn't so sure now. She had so little energy and was hot all the time. She was used to getting up at night to visit the bathroom and could overlook that, but the night sweats were also taking their toll on her outlook. She couldn't remember the last time that she and her husband had sex. When they did start cuddling, ripples of searing heat that led to profuse sweating arrived, which was a turn off for both of them. The only place they could have sex was in the shower, but that had it own set of issues. She didn't have the energy to try to figure that out, too.

Lena was drinking more and more coffee to stay awake and hadn't felt like herself in a while. She forced herself to smile and nod and listen to other moms complain about their kids, when she just felt like going home and taking a nap. She tried black cohosh, a medicinal herb, which worked for a few weeks, but when her symptoms returned, she made an appointment to see me. As we discussed the various options for treating her hot flashes, Lena bristled at the idea of using an antidepressant to treat them. "I'm not depressed," she said. "Since this is a hormonal change, how about we try hormones?" Lena's mom had taken Premarin for years and hadn't had any issues with it, so she was interested in an oral estrogen pill. She didn't need any added progesterone because of her hysterectomy a few years earlier for growing fibroids.

Lena was interested in the reports from the Kronos Early Estrogen and Progesterone Study (KEEPS) and was encouraged by the findings that younger, healthier women who didn't have high blood pressure or underlying heart disease seemed to have fewer serious side effects than women who were higher risk to begin with. She began taking a low dose of oral estrogen and felt better within a week. She could deal with one hot flash every few days and never missed the racing heart or roaring in her ears. As an added benefit, she didn't have to switch to iced coffee and was sleeping better at night.

Gradually her moods improved and she felt more like participating in her kids' activities, with plenty of energy left at the end of each day for the hot and sexy Saturday nights with her husband. Date nights were a lot more fun now that she could cuddle without feeling like she was in a steam room.

THE NITTY-GRITTY ON HORMONES

As women take the ride on the hormonal roller coaster of perimenopause and menopause, their estrogen levels decline, leading to all sorts of changes in virtually every aspect of their lives, from how their skin looks to how much interest and enjoyment they have in sex. A drop in estrogen can also bring hot flashes, night sweats, and vaginal dryness (see Chapter 6).

The current thinking is, if women want to use hormones, they should start as close to menopause as possible—in other words, when they're symptomatic. They should use the lowest effective dose and discuss with their own healthcare provider how long they can continue to use hormones. Women who use estrogen will also need to use a progestin or progesterone to balance the effects of estrogen and decrease the risk of developing endometrial cancer in the lining of the uterus.

About ten years ago, virtually every woman over forty was urged to use estrogen and progesterone hormone treatment. They were told to stay on hormones well into their seventies, eighties, and beyond. Women and their practitioners were less aware of the risks and concentrated on the perceived benefits, from the elimination of hot flashes and night sweats, to better skin and a healthy sex drive. Then suddenly, in 2002, everything changed. The report of the findings of the Women's Health Initiative (WHI) study shocked many healthcare practitioners and led millions of women to stop using hormones.

The WHI study of over 160,000 women showed that the use of estrogen and progesterone increased the risk of blood clots, stroke, and breast cancer. It was a tectonic shift in the prevailing thought on menopausal treatment, though earlier studies had found similar associations. The uproar and fallout was immediate. Women felt betrayed and abruptly stopped their hormones. Healthcare providers and thought leaders had to rethink some of what they had previously believed and began looking into the research for more specific answers. There's much to criticize about the WHI, and much to learn. Here are some of the limitations of the WHI study:

- The women studied were only given Premarin or PremPro (a combination of Premarin with Provera).

- Many of the women studied were over sixty years of age.

- A significant number had other risk factors for stroke, including high blood pressure and smoking.

In the meantime, more evidence was accumulating that showed that after millions of women stopped their hormones in the wake of the WHI findings, breast cancer rates also dropped. Since the WHI, other smaller studies with fewer women have shown fewer risks in younger, healthier women using lower doses and different formulations, and compared using estrogen patches to taking oral pills.

It took years to pore over the data to see that it was probable that younger, healthy, nonsmoking women who didn't have high blood pressure were at less risk, but the die was already cast. Millions of women no longer trusted the pharmaceutical companies and refused to even consider any hormone treatment for their symptoms. Others turned to what they believed to be safer alternatives—compounded hormones that haven't been studied, so the risks are unknown. Though it's a confusing, tangled mess of information, there is a lot that we do know:

1. Estrogen remains the most effective treatment for hot flashes and night sweats. Nothing compares to how much better women feel on every measurement of quality of life when they take estrogen. We know it works and it works well. The problem is that using estrogen is not completely risk free. There's no free lunch.

2. There are various formulations of estrogen available. Women can swallow a pill, use a patch, or rub a cream or gel onto their skin. Taking an estrogen pill versus using a patch, cream, or gel means that the estrogen is absorbed and metabolized differently, which can also influence the side effects and risks.

3. There are different options for obtaining bioidentical hormones to treat menopausal symptoms. Women can use prescriptions for bioidentical products that are FDA approved or they can visit compounding pharmacies, which may or may not use FDA-approved formulations.

4. We also know that using estrogen alone in women who have a uterus increases the risk of developing endometrial cancer (in the lining of the uterus). To prevent that, we have to balance estrogen by adding progesterone to the treatment, which further complicates the risk profile, because there are various kinds of progesterone and they, too, have their own risks.

Recently, the FDA approved a new and novel estrogen combination therapy to treat menopausal symptoms without using progesterone, and its associated risks, by substituting the progesterone with bazodoxifene. Bazodoxifene is a selective estrogen receptor modulator (SERM) that provides estrogen-like protection on some tissues but acts as an estrogen blocker on other tissues. This new combination of Premarin (conjugated equine estrogen) and bazodoxifene (brand name Duavee) was approved by the FDA in the fall of 2013 and is now available.

5. I think a lot of the confusion about hormonal treatments comes from people trying to make sense of less-than-perfect studies and looking for the safest ways to use the most effective treatment. There are too many different types of hormones, subtypes, subcategories, ways of using them, and differing molecules. Each has their own characteristics, and it's hard to generalize from one to another in terms of safety because the research doesn't compare them all head to head. In addition, the newer studies are looking at hundreds of women, not thousands of women.

Sex Drive and Hormone Treatments

Though there's no consensus on whether using hormones for hot flashes and night sweats improves sex drive, libido, and sexual response, still many women find that they're more interested in sex after starting hormone treatment. Whether it's the improved sleep or the hormonal influences on arousal, women have been pleasantly surprised by the return of their sex drive. The KEEPS trial also found that women on both low-dose oral estrogen and transdermal estrogen enjoyed more lubrication and less pain. There were also significant improvements in desire and arousal for the women on transdermal estrogen.

Breast Cancer and Hormone Treatments

Here's something else to consider. We've seen from many studies that the use of estrogens has been associated with an increased risk of breast cancer. It's not because estrogen causes normal, healthy breast cells to suddenly change and become cancerous, but they may contribute to accelerated growth of a small cancer that's already there and too small to be detected. Most of the breast cancers that were seen in the WHI study were found in the first three years of the study. It's thought that because breast cancers typically take more than five years to develop into something that can be detected, the estrogen use didn't start the process but instead may have caused the cancer to grow faster.

When we talk about estrogens and breast cancer, I want to make one important distinction: Using estrogens in doses that are high enough to treat hot flashes and night sweats is different from using much smaller doses to treat vaginal dryness. The use of small amounts of estrogen in the vagina has *not* been associated with breast cancer. There were other confusing findings from the WHI. One that was lost in translation with all of the brouhaha over hormones—and that sparked even more questions —was that for women who used estrogen alone, there was a slightly *decreased* likelihood of breast cancer. It wasn't statistically significant, because the numbers of women who were studied were so small, but this finding did raise a few eyebrows. This was also seen in the Nurses Health Study, but only for those women who used estrogen for less than ten years. Could it also be that the type of progesterone is a factor in the risk for breast cancer?

Putting Risk into Context

For the most part, the following statements are true: If you brush and floss your teeth, you're more likely to keep them. If you wear your safety belt, you're less likely to be injured in a crash. Still, for all these actions, and for a million more, doing all the right things doesn't mean that you're completely safe and have eliminated all risk; it just means that you're *less likely* to experience a pitfall or have an illness, injury, or condition.

One of the other maddening aspects women encounter when trying to decide whether to use hormones is the confusing way risks are communicated. In the WHI study, the risks for heart disease were different depending upon the ages of the women studied, how long they took the medication, and the risk factors they had prior to starting hormones.

Although there is an increased risk of heart disease, blood clots that can lead to a stroke or pulmonary embolism, and breast cancer when using estrogen and progesterone, these serious risks are somewhat rare.

For every 100 women who *do not* use hormones:

- 2 women will develop heart disease

- 2 others will have a stroke

- 2 will develop a pulmonary embolism (blood clot in the lung)

- 2 will develop breast cancer

For the women who *do* use hormones:

- 3 will develop heart disease

- 3 others will have a stroke

- 3 will develop a pulmonary embolism (blood clot in the lung)

- 3 will develop breast cancer

That means that for each of these very serious risks, in the Women's Health Initiative there was 1 extra woman in 100 who had one of these serious side effects. Communicated in a different way, when considering 10,000 woman-years, in women who took a combination of estrogen and progesterone, there were:

- 7 more cardiovascular events

- 8 more strokes

- 8 more clots in the lungs (pulmonary embolisms)

- 8 more breast cancers

- 6 fewer colorectal cancers

- 5 fewer hip fractures

. . . .

Nurse Barb's Quick Facts About Hormones

- Estrogen is available in many FDA-approved formulations in natural, synthetic, and bioidentical options.

- Estrogen works effectively to reduce hot flashes and night sweats for the majority of women who use it.

- Women with a uterus must use progesterone to decrease the effects estrogen can have on the endometrial (uterine) lining and therefore decrease the risk of overgrowth of the lining that, in rare cases, can lead to cancer of the endometrium.

- Estrogen that comes as a transdermal patch, cream, or gel appears to have *less* risk of blood clots than the oral estrogen tablets or pills.

- Bioidentical hormones can be found in prescription medications that are FDA approved.

- Women do not have to rely only on compounded estrogens if they are looking for a bioidentical formulation.

- Compounding pharmacies offer a variety of estrogen formulations. Some use combinations of estrogens, such as estradiol, estrone, and estriol. Some of these combinations are not FDA approved.

- All hormone treatments for hot flashes and night sweats, including compounded and FDA-approved formulations for menopause, may carry an increased risk of breast cancer.

- Using vaginal estrogen to treat dryness does not appear to increase the risk of breast cancer.

- Recent evidence from the Kronos Early Estrogen Prevention Study (KEEPS) found that younger women—those who start hormones in their early fifties—have fewer cardiovascular risks than women who start hormones in their sixties.

- Women should not start hormones if they are more than ten years from their last menstrual period.

- Synthetic progestins are different from micronized progesterone (Prometrium).

- There seems to be less risk of breast cancer and blood clots with micronized progesterone (Prometrium) than with Provera.

- A new preparation, DUAVEE, uses Premarin (a conjugated equine estrogen) plus bazodoxifene (a selective estrogen receptor modulator or SERM), instead of progesterone, to decrease estrogen's effects on the uterine lining. This is a novel approach that combines the proven hot flash and night sweat reductions of Premarin with a SERM that has estrogen-like effects on some tissues and antiestrogen effects on other tissues. This preparation was studied for three years in over 900 women and no increased risk of breast cancer was reported.

· ·

Nurse Barb's Smart Hormone Tips

- Do try nonhormonal remedies first to see if you can control your symptoms without incurring any risk no matter how remote or rare.

- Consider a transdermal estrogen formulation instead of oral preparations to mitigate the first-pass effects in the liver that can lead to changes in cholesterol values and the development of atherosclerosis and heart disease.

- Start with the lowest dose and slowly work your way up if necessary to control symptoms.

- Use the lowest effective dose for the least amount of time necessary.

- Before starting any hormone treatment, have your cholesterol and blood pressure checked and try other options if you're already at higher risk for heart disease or stroke.

- I don't recommend menopausal hormone use for women who smoke; it's too risky.

- Have yearly mammograms and automated breast ultrasound if you have dense breasts.

- Don't start hormone treatment if it's been more than ten years since your last period.

- Do discuss updates in research at your annual exam.

- If you decide to stop using hormones, wean off slowly to reduce the onset of severe hot flashes and night sweats.

- If your hot flashes are gone, but you still have vaginal dryness, ask your provider about a vaginal estrogen preparation to also use at the same time.

- If you have completely eradicated your hot flashes and night sweats, consider going to an even lower dose of estrogen.

MAKING A DECISION ABOUT HORMONE TREATMENT

Not every woman has debilitating hot flashes and night sweats. Some of those lucky women will sleep through the night and not wake in a hot, clammy sweat. Some will not have hot flashes that soak through clothes and leave beads of perspiration dripping from their foreheads. And yet, there are millions of women who do have such severe hot flashes and night sweats that they'll consider doing anything, because they want their lives back and are willing to accept the risks that accompany treatment options.

Though the primary reason most women use hormones is not to improve sexuality, it can be a happy byproduct and provides for a significant improvement in the quality of life. Since most of us will live an additional thirty to forty years after menopause, the promise of an active and healthy sex life is a benefit that is often overlooked when women are making choices about treatments.

For many women even a slight risk is too much; for others, the benefits of using estrogen and hormones far outweigh the slight and yet serious risks. When considering whether to use hormone treatments for menopause, it's best to take time with your healthcare provider and develop an individualized plan together. Use the lowest effective dose and stay up to date about newer options and research findings. Every year at your annual exam, it's a good idea to review any new research findings and the implications those might have in your own life. If you do decide to use hormones, use the lowest dose that helps your symptoms.

1 1

Getting the Skinny on Bioidentical Hormones and Compounded Hormones

I like the idea of using natural ingredients. I also like the idea of using bioidentical hormones. In fact, I prescribe FDA-approved formulations of bioidentical hormones to my patients. And yet, there is so much confusion among both women and healthcare practitioners about bioidentical hormones—whether they are natural and where they are available. Because of the confusion, I'd like to clarify a few myths and misconceptions.

After the Women's Health Initiative (WHI) study results showed that using the prescription hormones Premarin and PremPro, a combination of Premarin and Provera, were linked to serious health risks, many women decided to abandon all hormones available from pharmaceutical companies. Even though Premarin is derived from a natural source, the serious risks associated with long-term use caused many women and practitioners to rethink all hormone treatments in menopause. Before this study was reported, hormones were given out freely to millions of women without understanding the risks. Understandably, after the results were reported, women felt betrayed and became more skeptical of claims by pharmaceutical companies. Almost overnight, millions of women abruptly stopped using their hormones, and many of them started having severe hot flashes and night sweats. This left women and their healthcare practitioners in a quandary. Everyone seemed to be searching for safer options and looked to bioidentical hormones as a possible solution.

Many people reasoned that our bodies would probably react better to molecules that were *identical* to what our own bodies produced. It seems logical to avoid hormones that are different, which people thought might have led to the complications and risks seen in the WHI study. Around the same time celebrities were sharing their discoveries about compounded bioidentical hormones with the public in best-selling books.

Before the WHI study, few people had heard the term *bioidentical,* and now suddenly everyone wanted these types of hormones and the only place that seemed to have any idea about these hormones were compounding and specialty pharmacies. Overnight, the words *bioidentical* and *compounded* became synonymous. Many people still believe that the *only* source of bioidentical hormones is from compounding pharmacies; however, there are bioidentical estrogen and progesterone formulations that are FDA-approved, have research that outlines the risks and benefits, and are available from any pharmacy with a prescription.

Another factor that fuels the confusion is that many women distrust big pharmaceutical companies. We have seen too many drug recalls and read too many studies that show serious side effects. Women left Premarin and PremPro and other formulations behind because they were skeptical of marketing claims from all the big pharmaceutical companies and instead flocked to compounding pharmacies to get what they perceived as safer hormonal preparations to relieve their symptoms.

There were several problems with this thinking. First, there wasn't any research that showed that any bioidenticals from any source, regular or specialty pharmacy, were safer. Also, many natural products were not bioidentical. In addition, compounding pharmacies weren't the only source of bioidentical hormones. Finally, the compounding pharmacies were using different types of estrogens, estradiol, estrone, and estriol (see Chapter 6) and mixing them together. These formulations have not been adequately studied in menopausal women, which means that we don't know if they are safer or carry more risks. We just don't know because those studies haven't been done and there are no plans to look at those formulations for safety concerns.

Women want effective safe hormonal preparations, and compounding pharmacies seemed to be offering just that. Unfortunately, many of the claims that are made can't be backed up with actual research, which prevented them from gaining FDA approval. Are you confused yet? I know my patients are. And yet, we know a lot more now than we did a few years ago. What we've found may reassure you. There are bioidentical hormone preparations that have been studied for both their effectiveness and safety. These are available at your local pharmacy with a prescription. We also know that some women don't tolerate these prescription medications and may need to have a compounding pharmacy produce a different formulation for them.

I have patients who prefer the bioidentical estradiol gel from the compounding pharmacy, and because estradiol has been studied for it's effectiveness and safety, I'm comfortable with that. I'm not comfortable recommending other compounded formulations that use combinations of various estrogens and/or progestins because the safety hasn't been adequately studied.

Let me give you a little bit more context to help understand natural, bioidentical, and compounded hormones. Let's start with the term "natural hormones." They seem somehow safer. Honestly, I don't think about the process behind the manufacturing of natural ingredients. I completely skip over what's actually involved in processing all of these "natural" products. I don't know about you, but when I see the word "natural" associated with hormones, I envision a woman with long flowing hair in a embroidered cotton blouse and loose skirt in a lovely field of sunflowers. She has a pleasant smile that emanates from within her peaceful and serene life of daily yoga and herb gathering. The woven basket on her arm is filled with aromatic herbs and lavender tied with a ribbon. That's what I picture when I think of "natural" products.

The truth is, truckloads of ingredients or drums filled with the components are delivered onto conveyor belts that eventually wind up in the little pill or patch that I'm using. I see the word "natural" and I think of the lady in the field, crushing all those herbs by hand, and then magically they appear in the tube or the bottle of my "natural" remedies in beautiful packaging that reassures me of the safety and efficacy.

The reality though is quite different. All of the natural, and yes, even the bioidentical and compounded products available, while derived from natural ingredients like yams and soy, are actually processed in large sterile labs the size of several football fields, where lots of people in white bunny suits and goggles oversee the production process. It's overwhelming for me, too. I don't like to think about the actual process involved in making medications, but there you have it. It's big business no matter what you're using, what soothing colors are on the label, or what the model on the ads looks like in the magazines.

In our minds, we might believe that an estrogen derived from a natural source such as a wild yam or an organic soybean is better for us than one produced in a test tube. And yet, according to many experts and the FDA, estrogen is estrogen is estrogen, meaning that your cells really don't care where your estrogen comes from, whether it's a lab in Arkansas or derived from a plant in Katmandu that is then sent to a lab somewhere for final processing. If the molecule and the way it's delivered to your cells is the same, your body will use it the same way and the risks will be the same. Really? Yes. So we all have to assume that any estrogen that we're using to eliminate those bothersome hot flashes and night sweats no matter where it comes from has the same risks. But wait, aren't there some differences? Okay, maybe.

There Might Be Some Differences

Is all estrogen the same? Maybe not. Notice I mentioned two important differences: the molecule itself and the way it gets into your body. These are the keys to all the confusion about bioidentical, synthetic, and natural hormones and may make a big difference in their safety. These principles also apply for progesterone.

The key here is that there are different estrogen molecules available to you. Some are natural, some are synthetic, and some are bioidentical. Some are derived from a natural source *and* are synthetic. Some are synthetic *and* bioidentical at the same time; some are natural *and* bioidentical. That means you might be using a bioidentical hormone that starts in a lab, is synthetic, or made in a test tube, and not from a natural source. There are bioidentical hormones that are FDA approved, have research behind them, and are available by prescription. There are also bioidentical compounded hormones that have limited safety data, are not FDA approved, and are only available from a compounding pharmacy. Still confused?

Estrogen can be:	Estrogen is available as:
Synthetic	Pills
Natural	Patches
Bioidentical	Creams
FDA approved	Sprays
Compounded with FDA approval	Gels
Compounded without FDA approval	Combined with progesterone

Progesterone can be:

Synthetic	Bioidentical

Finding the best options for treating hot flashes and night sweats can be challenging when there is so much confusing information out there vying for our attention. I'd like you to meet two of my patients, Beth and Ariana, who wanted to use bioidentical hormones for relief.

BETH'S STORY

As a self-proclaimed night owl, Beth was an ICU nurse who had seen every life-and-death situation in her twenty years working the night shift. She was the kind of calm, cool professional everyone counted on in a crisis. No situation, no matter how chaotic, ever seemed to faze this steady rock that everyone from patients and families to other hospital staff relied upon. Beth had been my patient for over ten years. I knew from the way she asked questions and processed information that she was a strong and capable woman who could handle anything.

When Beth came in after six months of wildly irregular periods, some surprising mood swings, and debilitating hot flashes that occurred day and night, I was surprised by how she looked and what she said.

"I feel like I'm moving in slow motion through a steam room. I'm so hot all the time, I can't function and I'm freaked out by all the crying," she explained. "In my job, I can't stop everything and run to the bathroom for

a quick cry, but these last few months, my emotions are all over the map. I've never been a crier. I don't have a lot of respect for criers, but now, guess what? I'm a crier. I don't like it. Help me make this all stop!" she was half pleading, half demanding.

Beth had done her research. She went to conferences and read journal articles searching for the best options for overwhelming hot flashes that left her drained and depressed. Looking at the risks of heart disease, blood clots, and breast cancer, and weighing them against her quality of life, Beth reasoned that she was low risk for the more serious side effects. She knew from experience that anything could happen to anyone at anytime, but with her low cholesterol levels, normal blood pressure, and no family history of breast cancer, she was in a low-risk group. She wanted to use bioidentical hormones for both estrogen and progesterone and wanted to know her options.

Beth felt more comfortable staying with FDA-approved medications. She liked knowing that there was evidence to support the claims and the adverse events and felt more comfortable with bioidentical preparations. She decided to use a transdermal estrogen patch that she'd change twice each week. Because the only bioidentical progesterone available was oral, she'd also take an oral Prometrium capsule each morning when she ended her night shift and went to sleep.

Within a few weeks, Beth called to say that the crying had virtually stopped and that she was feeling cool again. "It's such a relief," she explained. "I feel like my old self again, and I can handle anything that life throws my way." Beth has been on these preparations for several years. Each year we review the data and she decides to continue.

ARIANA'S STORY

Ariana came to see me after finding a worrisome lump in her left breast. She was fifty-six, and as a dance instructor, she was in superb health. She wasn't too worried about breast cancer, she explained, as she had no family history and had been using bioidentical hormones for the last two years. She obtained them from a compounding pharmacy after going to a seminar on natural hormones.

I felt my own heart rate speed up as I palpated the kumquat-sized lump in her breast that was firmly attached to her chest wall. Luckily, I couldn't feel any enlarged lymph nodes. After arranging an immediate diagnostic mammogram that afternoon, we talked for a few minutes. I explained that while 90 percent of lumps turn out to be benign and noncancerous, there was still a chance that this could be more worrisome, and she'd need further evaluation.

Later the radiologist called to discuss the findings. My heart sank. The lump was highly suspicious for breast cancer. I arranged an appointment for Ariana the next day with a breast specialist who did a needle biopsy. A few days later, she received the diagnosis: the lump was breast cancer and she'd need to make some decisions about the next steps.

Understandably overwhelmed, Ariana came to see me after visiting with four other healthcare practitioners. She had so many conflicting feelings, ranging from shock and anger to sadness and fear, that she was immobilized. She was left with more questions than answers.

"I thought I was safe," she said. "I thought I was doing all the right things. I purposely didn't use the hormones from pharmaceutical companies; that's why I went with compounded, natural bioidenticals. I don't understand how this could have happened to me. It's like a betrayal." As I listened to Ariana, I felt a lot of sympathy for her. She was like many women who hear that a particular remedy is "more natural" and then leap to the conclusion that because it's natural or bioidentical that it's completely risk free.

At the time that she obtained her compounded hormones, the FDA hadn't mandated that there be any warnings listed on the medications. Like millions of women, Ariana assumed that natural was safer.

It's impossible to know if Ariana would have developed breast cancer whether she had been on hormones or not. Would it have mattered if she was on nothing, took a pharmaceutical hormone preparation, or took her compounded formulations? Since breast cancers can take over five years to develop, and she was only using bioidentical hormones for two years, if anything, they probably helped accelerate the growth of a breast cancer that was already there and may have contributed to her feeling it earlier than she would have had she not been on hormones.

Ariana eventually decided to have a lumpectomy, radiation, and tamox-

ifen. She used gabapentin for the night sweats that resulted from her tamoxifen use and has been cancer free for over five years.

BREAST CANCER AND MENOPAUSAL HORMONES

My mother was diagnosed with breast cancer at age thirty-two and luckily lived a long and healthy life after her mastectomy. I've also cared for many women who have had breast cancer. Many did not use any hormones for their hot flashes and night sweats, and many did. So what's the risk? It's important to remember that all women are at risk for breast cancer. In our lifetime, one in eight women will have breast cancer, the majority of whom will be over fifty years of age when they are diagnosed.

Some of us are a little bit more likely to develop breast cancer. Those of us with a strong family history of one or more close relatives, a mother or sisters, with breast cancer are at higher risk. We now know that genetic mutations with BRCA1 or BRCA2 genes, or other variants, increase the likelihood of developing breast and ovarian cancer.

Still, there are many more women with no family history and nothing in their life or lifestyle that predicts that they'll develop breast cancer, and yet they get diagnosed every year. It can be extremely jarring and impossible to imagine that the diagnosis is real, especially when these women are healthy, eat right, drink very little alcohol, and exercise regularly. These are women who play by the rules and do everything they're supposed to do. All of this mitigates and reduces risks but doesn't completely eliminate them.

When it comes to women who use hormones to treat hot flashes and night sweats, compared to women who don't use hormones, some women in both groups will develop breast cancer. As yet, we don't have any data on the rates of breast cancer in women on compounded hormones, which are made with a combination of estrogens and may include estrone and or estriol. It's impossible to know whether one, two, or all three of these estrogens are associated with an increased risk of breast cancer. We don't know if it's better, worse, or the same for women who don't use hormones or who use FDA-approved pharmaceutical options, or for women who use compounded hormones. The studies haven't been done. The jury is still out. Ariana assumed that, because she used a bioidentical formulation from a specialty compounding pharmacy, she was immunized from the risk of breast cancer, but unfortunately that wasn't the case. It's also important that all women who use estrogen to treat their menopausal symptoms, but not the vaginal preparations, be informed of the increased risk of breast cancer.

Is Progesterone a Factor in Breast Cancer?

This is an important question and here's why. One finding from the WHI that was lost in translation with the brouhaha over hormones was that, for women who used estrogen alone without taking progestins, there was a slightly *decreased* likelihood of breast cancer. It wasn't statistically significant, because the numbers of women studied were small, but this finding did raise a few eyebrows. This same trend was also seen in the Nurses Health Study, but only for women who used estrogen for less than ten years. Is it possible that when it comes to hormone treatment and breast cancer, at least in the first few years after menopause, the type of progesterone is a factor in breast cancer risk? The jury is still out on this because the recent studies have only looked at very small numbers of women.

Progesterone Is Different from Progestins

When researchers and clinicians try to individualize the recommendations for hormone treatments for women, we're trying to minimize the woman's risk of developing breast cancer. We have to rely on the available research, while also relieving symptoms. One of the issues in terms of risk of breast cancer is what influence progesterone has.

There's a lot of confusion about the difference between progesterone and progestins. Progesterone is the molecule that our bodies make. Until relatively recently, there weren't any formulations of progesterone that were both identical to what our bodies make and able to be absorbed orally. Synthetic progestins were created that could be absorbed and converted to progesterone. But now there is Prometrium, which is a micronized oral progesterone, able to be absorbed orally, which is identical to what our bodies make—in other words, "bioidentical." It's not advised for women with a peanut allergy as it's made with peanut oil.

In the European E3N-EPIC study (the French component of the European Prospective Investigation into Cancer and Nutrition), 50,000 women on various progestins were followed for approximately six years. This study found that there was no increased risk of blood clots or breast cancer in women on Prometrium. In fact, their risk of blood clots and breast cancer were the same as women who were not using any hormones. This study and the recent data from the KEEPS trial, which also used Prometrium, has led many clinicians to switch their patients from synthetic progestins to the micronized oral bioidentical, Prometrium. This table lists the various progestin formulations available.

* *

Synthetic Progestins Found in Hormone Formulations:

Medroxyprogesterone acetate: found in PremPro, PremPhase, Cycrin, and Amen

Norethindrone acetate: found in Activella, Aygestin, Combipatch, and FemHRT

Norgestimate: found in Ortho Prefest

Bioidentical Progesterone: Prometrium

* *

THE NITTY-GRITTY ON BIOIDENTICAL HORMONES & COMPOUNDED HORMONES

Prior to 2002, when the Women's Health Initiative (WHI) study results revealed serious risks from taking menopausal hormone treatment, very few women had heard the term "bioidentical." Then suddenly overnight, bioidentical hormones became a newsworthy sensation as millions of women searched for alternatives that would be safer than the pharmaceutical hormone preparations used in the study. (See Appendix on page 259.)

When we talk about using estrogen to treat menopausal symptoms, we have to remember that there are many forms of estrogen. Estradiol is one of the "bioidentical" estrogen hormones made by our ovaries. It's the one that's found in menopausal hormonal treatments. There are many

FDA-approved bioidentical hormonal preparations that contain estradiol. These are available as a pill that's taken by mouth or as a transdermal preparation using a patch, gel, cream, or vaginal ring.

· ·

List of FDA-Approved Bioidentical Estrogens

Oral tablets

Estrace

Angeliq (has bioidentical estrogen and a synthetic progestin, drospirenone)

Patch

Alora	Estraderm	Vivelle-Dot
Climara	Esclim	

Gels, Creams, Sprays

Divigel	EstroGel	Evamist
Elestrin	Estrasorb	

Vaginal preparations

Estring	Femring	Vagifem

Compounded Bioidenticals that are FDA approved

Estradiol

Compounded Bioidenticals that are not FDA approved

Bi-Est	Tri-Est

· ·

Oral Bioidentical Estrogens Versus Bioidentical Transdermals?

Another question that comes up with bioidentical hormones is should I take them by mouth or use them on my skin as a transdermal. Transdermal preparations simply mean that the hormones are absorbed into our bodies through our skin from a cream, gel, patch, or spray. The bottom line is no matter what kind of oral estrogen is used, there's an increased risk of developing dangerous blood clots. This is because oral medications must first undergo metabolism by the liver. When estrogen is applied directly to the skin, in the form of a patch, gel, cream, or mist, there is no "first-pass" effect in the liver, which decreases but may not completely eliminate the risk of blood clots. Many providers are switching their patients away from oral estrogens and over to transdermal estrogens.

Compounded Hormones

In the quest for effective hormonal alternatives to pharmaceutical preparations with known benefits and serious adverse effects, many women turned to compounded preparations because they were thought to be safer. Many women and many clinicians used the terms natural, bio-identical, and compounded to mean the same thing. And though many women reasoned that, because these hormones were compounded, they must somehow be safer, there was no evidence or research supporting these hopes. Many of my patients assumed that compounded hormones were the only source of bioidentical hormones and were safer alternatives to FDA-approved pharmaceutical options. With compounding pharmacies using words like "natural" and "bioidentical" to promote these remedies, the confusion was only magnified.

Compounded hormones use the same bioidentical estrogen hormones that we produce in our bodies: estriol, estrone, and estradiol (see Chapter 6).

I understand the thinking behind using compounded bioidentical hormones. Estriol and estrone are less potent than estradiol, so it would seem reasonable to assume that they'd be a safer alternative to using estradiol. And since estrone is the most prevalent hormone in menopause, it also seems like the logical choice to replace what's lost. Unfortunately, there just isn't enough research on large numbers of women over many years to back up any of the safety claims that are made. We don't know if using compounded hormones are a safe alternative to conventional hormone treatment. We don't know if they carry the same, fewer, or more risks. We just don't know, and it's unwise to assume that just because they're compounded or that they come from a "natural source" that they are somehow safer.

I have no doubt that these formulations are very effective at decreasing hot flashes and night sweats. I know that many of my patients have been very happy with these formulations and many have been on them for years without any adverse effects or serious side effects. I also have patients who react to various ingredients in pharmaceutical preparations and need a compounded formulation. For example, some women who are allergic to peanuts and can't take Prometrium use a compounded progesterone instead.

For women like Ariana, who develop serious side effects from using compounded hormones, it's impossible to know if they would have had those same events on a different hormone preparation or on no hormones. What is important to understand is that compounded formulations are still hormones, and all hormones carry risks. We can't assume that because they are made with less potent estrogens that they are automatically safer.

Salivary Testing for Hormone Levels

Many practitioners who recommend compounded bioidentical hormones utilize salivary testing to determine hormone levels. To say that this is controversial would be an enormous understatement. Providers are either in one camp or another, and there isn't any middle ground. Where does that leave patients? They're scratching their heads in confusion. From the research I've done and the experts I've spoken to, it's my belief and the position of the North American Menopause Society (NAMS) that salivary testing isn't of any value, at least for estradiol levels.

I haven't seen any compelling evidence that the results from salivary testing correlate with blood levels or with women's symptoms. We know that estrogen levels can vary widely from hour to hour and from day to day and this is even more apparent in salivary testing. It's also a concern that there aren't any independent laboratories that have validated the normal range of estrogen and progesterone levels in saliva. I prefer to recommend treatments based on patient's symptoms.

What's in Compounded Hormones?

Compounded hormones use two or more of the same bioidentical estrogen hormones that we produce in our bodies: estriol, estrone, and estradiol.

ESTRIOL is the hormone most prevalent in pregnancy. It's 1/80th as potent as estradiol. This is the major component in compounded hormones. It's considered the weakest estrogen. There isn't a lot of safety data on estriol and its risks; therefore, it's not approved by the FDA.

ESTRONE is the hormone most prevalent in women during menopause and is converted to estradiol. It's about 1/10th as potent as estradiol. There isn't a lot of research on estrone either, and that's why it's not approved by the FDA.

ESTRADIOL is the most potent estrogen. Of the three estrogens in compounded hormones, only estradiol has been studied enough to gain FDA approval and is available in a variety of prescription medications.

The two most common compounded estrogen therapies are Bi-Est and Tri-Est.

BI-EST contains estriol and estradiol. There are various percentages of each hormone in each prescription, which can be adjusted. Some of the most common formulations of Bi-Est are:

- Bi-Est 80/20: Estriol 80%, Estradiol 20%

- Bi-Est 50/50: Estriol 50%, Estradiol 50%

TRI-EST contains estriol, estrone, and estradiol. This formulation is used much less now, as many practitioners prefer not to add estrone to the compounded mixture because menopausal women already have quite a bit of it circulating in their system. There are various percentages of each hormone in each prescription, which can be adjusted. Some of the most common formulations of Tri-Est are:

- Tri-Est 90/5/5: Estriol 90%, Estrone 5%, Estradiol 5%

- Tri-Est 80/10/10: Estriol 80%, Estrone 10%, Estradiol 10%

- Tri-Est 60/20/20: Estriol 60%, Estrone 20%, Estradiol 20%

These are available in a variety of different delivery systems, including creams, tinctures, capsules, troches (lozenges), pellets, or vaginal suppositories.

Compounded Progesterone

Compounding pharmacies may also provide progesterone cream that is derived from a botanical source, wild Mexican yams. These are available as capsules, creams, troches (lozenges), or vaginal suppositories. Just as compounded estrogens haven't been studied, neither have compounded progesterones. Many clinicians are concerned about whether the amounts of progesterone in these medications are sufficient, and about whether the body can absorb them in the amounts required to balance the effects of the compounded estrogens. There have been case reports in Australia of endometrial cancer associated with compounded progesterones.

Nurse Barb's Hot Hormone Tips

- Use your symptoms as your guide to determine whether your dose of hormones is right for you. If you're still having hot flashes and night sweats, you may need more.

- If you have completely eradicated your hot flashes and night sweats, consider going to a lower dose of estrogen.

- If you're interested in bioidentical hormones, do consider ones that are FDA approved as there is good safety data behind these products that identifies possible risks.

- If you decide to use compounded bioidentical estrogen formulations, you have to assume that the risks of breast cancer are the same as those available with prescription formulations.

- A specialty compounding pharmacy can provide estradiol, which has good safety data and is FDA approved.

- Avoid starting hormones if you are more than ten years from your last period.

- Have cholesterol and blood pressure checked before starting hormone treatment.

- Have a yearly mammogram and automated breast ultrasound if your breasts develop increased density.

- Use the presence or absence of hot flashes, night sweats, and other symptoms as your guide to whether your hormone levels are adequate.

- Don't rely on blood or saliva tests to check hormone levels; there's too much variability in results.

- Avoid the temptation to think that any compounded hormone treatment that has limited safety data is automatically safer than conventional treatments.

- Consider the safety data on low-dose oral estrogen and transdermal estrogen when making your decision.

- Consider using a bioidentical micronized progesterone preparation.

- If your hot flashes are gone, but you still have vaginal dryness, do ask your practitioner about a vaginal estrogen preparation.

REVIEWING YOUR OPTIONS

When considering whether to use hormone treatments—bioidentical, compounded, or synthetic—for menopause, it's best to take time with your healthcare provider and get an individualized plan. Remember, bioidentical hormones are available by prescription from any pharmacy as well as from compounding pharmacies. There are different ways for your body to absorb estrogens. You can use a pill, patch, cream, spray, gel, or vaginal ring. We know that estrogen works very well to eliminate hot flashes and night sweats, but there's no free lunch. There are some risks associated with using estrogen and progesterone. We're learning more about how to individualize hormone treatment based on a woman's symptoms, her age, her family, and medical history, and what is most bothersome to her. We also want to try to reduce the risks that we know come with this option. Yes, it's confusing and complicated. As with everything else in life, one size definitely doesn't fit all. Always get the information you need to make the best decisions for your health. No matter what you choose, start with the lowest effective dose, review your options every year at your annual exam, and stay up to date about options.

12

Losing the Meno Potbelly

I don't remember when or where I heard the term "meno potbelly" first, but I immediately recognized the brilliance of the term and now share it frequently with patients and friends. One day, I looked at myself in the mirror and was horrified to see that I, too, had developed a dreaded meno potbelly. I'm going to share with you the same strategies I use myself and recommend to my patients to not only lose it and stay fit but also to keep the meno potbelly at bay. These suggestions are all based on research and what really works to keep the weight off for good.

There are as many theories about menopausal weight distribution and weight gain as there are experts. Research supports what countless women have discovered for themselves: menopause brings with it a rapid accumulation of fat smack-dab at the waist.

Many experts believe that the shifting sands of declining hormone levels cause our bodies to redistribute fat from our arms, legs, and hips and plunk it down at our waists. Most of my patients believe that this seismic shift occurs overnight. In addition, lower estrogen levels and age-related changes all add up to a net decrease in lean muscle mass. Less muscle means that it's more difficult to burn the same amount of calories as we did in our twenties, thirties, and even five years previously. Women often complain that their diets are the same but their waistline is the only recipient of all the calories.

It's not as if all women at midlife suddenly start indulging every night in hot fudge brownie sundaes with whipped cream, or bags of salty potato chips, or both, thank you very much. No, despite being good, having salad with dressing on the side, and looking wistfully at the dessert menu, and then deciding to skip it, many women notice that their actual weight hasn't changed; the scale hasn't budged, but there's new bulging rolls of belly fat.

Some of us can't remember ever being "the skinny one." We fantasize about being able to easily glide into a size 6 or 8. For those of us who sometimes need heavy machinery just to pull the skinny jeans past our thighs, and would be thrilled not to have to lie on the floor just to zip them up, menopause can bring with it a surprise. We may finally have the satisfaction of seeing some of our thinner friends have just a small taste of what our lifelong reality has been. And yes, I'm going to admit it: This can be a very satisfying and smug experience. "Welcome to my world," we want to shout at their new struggles with a less-than-perfect body.

Secretly we're happy to see them in the same leaky rowboat with us. "Oh, you poor thing, you can't get into a size 8 anymore, really?" you say. "I'm lucky to squeeze into a size 12, hello?" "Don't even complain to me about not being able to wear a bikini. I haven't worn a bikini since preschool."

There's a perverse pleasure in seeing other women we envied for their flat stomachs and toned arms encounter our very own struggles with weight. Now, having said that, there's a lot we can learn from our thinner friends, so I'm going to encourage you not to get too complacent, snarky, and smug—or give up—because IT'S NEVER TOO LATE to get in better shape and lose the meno potbelly. As an added benefit, when you feel better about your body, your confidence and interest in sex are much more likely to increase as well. You can have a more hot and sexy menopause with a few less pounds.

The science behind how amazingly complicated our metabolism works can be daunting to understand. As it turns out, it's a lot more convoluted than simply calories in as food and calories out as energy. There are a myriad of hormones at work and intricate pathways that influence how much fat we store and how resistant it is to being shed. New research is looking at how the bacteria in our intestines determine whether to rev up our metabolism and burn those calories for fuel or store them as fat.

What most of my patients and friends want to know about weight loss is that they aren't the only ones who struggle with these issues. Virtually every woman on the planet thinks about her weight and how she looks in her clothes and whether she's exercising enough. I'd like to introduce you to three women who are just like you. Sam, Chris, and Nadia are all trying to get to a healthy weight without wiring their jaws shut or running marathons every weekend.

SAM'S STORY

Sam couldn't believe it. Her girlfriends said that this would happen, but she never really bought in to the idea. Instead, she pretended to agree, nodding her head and trying to be sympathetic of their plight. "There's no way I'm getting fat like that." She knew she was being mean. "But come on, how hard could it be to get to the gym?" she thought.

Sam was certain that her girlfriends were exaggerating about how much they exercised. They simply ate way too much. She had almost been stabbed by flying forks as her friends powered through the shared desserts at girls' night out. It was like watching sharks in a feeding frenzy whenever a chocolate lava cake was laid in the middle of a table full of women.

Sam was certain her friends had lost all their willpower as soon as they discovered the miracle of Spanx. And like every woman she knew, she was still kicking herself for not inventing them. But as she struggled to pull up her own Spanx over her expanding middle, she was still half convinced this was just bloating and a lingering effect from the Chinese takeout from a few nights back. "I think the dry cleaner is shrinking my pants," she said to her husband one morning on her way to work. He was smart enough to keep his mouth closed.

It seemed to Sam that the day after her fiftieth birthday, her body suddenly changed overnight without any notice or warning. It was like some terrible nightmare; her flat tummy was gone and in its place was a doughy, thick roll of fat. Sam had always exercised and watched what she ate. She wasn't eating more or exercising less. Nothing was different from what she had been doing for years. Sam was aghast at her reflection in the mirror; month after month, it never got thinner. She knew that, like her friends, she would have to make a few changes if she wanted to fit into her clothes again.

Sam decided to increase her exercise by adding a walk every evening, and she added weight training twice a week. She also increased her vegetable intake and switched from sandwiches to salads at lunch. It took three months, and the process was slow, but with a few simple changes, Sam lost most of the added flab at her midsection.

CHRIS'S STORY

Chris was a longtime patient who surprised me during her annual exam. She was scowling when I walked into the room. I heard the exam table paper crinkle as she shifted her weight. I hadn't seen her this angry in the years since I started caring for her. "What's going on with you?" I asked, smiling as I washed my hands.

"I can't believe that I'm so freaking fat," she blurted out. This was from a woman who always chose her words carefully. I'd never before heard her swear. Chris was used to being in control of her life and her body.

"I don't understand how I could have only gained five pounds in the last year. Your scale and my scale say five pounds, but I know it's more like twenty-five, and it's all right here." She jabbed her index finger at her midsection. "I'm paunchy. I've never been paunchy. All I can eat for lunch is baby freaking carrots and I'm still paunchy. I gave up wine, and I gave up chocolate. I gave up breakfast. I'm practically starving myself. I'm biking six hours on weekends and still, this!" The steam had evaporated from her eruption, but she was still fuming.

"Oh, and I'm really irritable all the time." She thought that training for a mini-triathlon would fix everything, because weight loss had always been easy for her with a little exercise, but even a grueling training schedule wasn't working. She got so discouraged after seeing a net loss of two pounds and a miniscule difference in her midsection that she gave up completely and ate whatever she wanted, which led to an even wider middle.

"I feel like my body is like an obstinate kid who won't give up a toy, no matter how much you reason with him." In a sense she was right. I asked Chris to keep a food and exercise diary for two weeks and then come in

to see me. She was surprised when I told her at the next visit that she was actually not eating enough, and her exercise wasn't consistent enough to help her lose weight. Chris skipped meals and ate so little that her body's energy production slowed down even with her exercising. Her body reacted as if she were starving herself and stopped burning as many calories to protect what weight she had. In addition, she was only doing aerobic activity and needed to add some resistance or weight training to build more muscle—the more lean muscle mass you have, the more calories you burn. I asked Chris to add more protein to her diet, to eat three small meals each day, and to add three high-protein snacks in between. Chris not only lost five pounds, she became a lot trimmer over several months. In addition, eating more frequently helped reduce her irritability from chronic hunger.

NADIA'S STORY

Nadia often looked in her refrigerator for the answers to her life's big questions. Why wasn't her husband more affectionate? Why was her daughter a little distant? Why couldn't she learn to say no to yet another volunteering opportunity? Why was she so tired? Rather than think about any of that, it was easier to go to the pantry for a bag of cookies that she could munch on mindlessly while watching Dancing with the Stars.

She was so busy that she didn't have time to exercise, and besides, she never really liked going to the gym because in truth, she felt too self-conscious in workout clothes. When Nadia came in for her annual physical, she wanted to know what she could do to drop thirty pounds in a week, just in time for her class reunion. She was only half joking when she asked, but I recognized the familiar request. "I need to jump-start my diet."

Nadia and every woman on the planet knows that it's impossible to lose thirty pounds in just one week before a reunion or big event, and yet we want to believe that there's a magic wand or new pill or special diet that will magically evaporate the pounds overnight.

I know this, because I also want to believe it. I want to be able to have a chocolate croissant every morning, a burger and fries for lunch, a pound of pasta for dinner, never exercise, and still be healthy and thin.

When I talked about this with Nadia, she nodded her head. "I know exactly what you mean," she said. "I should be able to eat what I want and not gain any weight. Why should I deprive myself? It's not fair." Nadia put into words what many of us think. "Why me?" Why should I have to restrict my intake when there's all this great food around all the time? And here's what I tell my patients, which has helped many of them move past the unrealistic expectations and the anger toward becoming more mindful of the choices we make:

I feel your pain. You're not alone in this. You haven't been singled out. I'm right there with you, too! It may surprise you to learn that only 3 percent of people on the planet are born with the thin gene and can eat whatever they like and never gain an ounce. Personally, I think that those people are mutants or aliens or something, but they're definitely not the norm. So, welcome to the club! That means that you're like 97 percent of the rest of us, who cannot eat anything we want and never gain weight. Virtually everyone you meet also has to make choices about what to eat and what to avoid.

Nadia told me later that knowing that just about everyone had the same struggles was helpful to her. She could now look around a restaurant with new eyes, noticing all the people eating salads and skipping desserts. She no longer focused on what she couldn't do, but on what she could do and started using words like, "I won't eat this," instead of, "I can't eat this."

As Nadia developed more awareness of the emotional triggers that led her to overeat, she found that food was one way she was nurturing herself and numbing herself from some uncomfortable feelings.

THE NITTY-GRITTY ON THE MENO POTBELLY

Many experts believe that the hormonal changes that lead to the meno potbelly and a woman's visible change in weight distribution also have an indirect effect on how we burn calories and metabolize carbohydrates. Studies haven't shown a direct correlation between the drop in hormone levels in menopause and insulin resistance, but they have shown that accumulation of fat at the midsection is associated with increased insulin resistance, increased hunger, and a change in carbohydrate metabolism.

So while there isn't a direct line from lower estrogen levels to insulin resistance, there may well be a more circuitous route that leads to the same destination: elastic waistbands.

Here's how I explain the meno potbelly to my patients:

- As we age, we naturally lose lean muscle mass.

- Ounce per ounce and pound per pound, lean muscle burns more calories for fuel than other tissue.

- The same number of calories taken in will now will produce a little extra fat, which gets deposited in the arms, hips, thighs, and midsection.

- The same amount of fat doesn't weigh as much as muscle or the water in our bodies.

- Women can eat the same number of calories, be losing muscle mass and replacing it with fat, which weighs less, so the scale doesn't change, and yet there's a greater percentage of fat than previously and a reduced percentage of muscle.

- Around menopause, some of the excess fat deposited around the body decides to have a big family reunion at the waist. So seemingly overnight, women wake up to a meno potbelly.

- The more fat that's deposited at the midsection, the more likely it is that your body isn't metabolizing carbohydrates as efficiently, which can lead to insulin resistance and diabetes.

- As fat accumulates in the midsection, something even more insidious occurs: that fat sends out more of the hormone ghrelin to the brain, which acts to increase appetite.

- What seems to be a sudden occurrence is actually a few years in the making.

- Don't be discouraged. By understanding the mechanics behind the meno potbelly, you can lose weight and be healthier by making better choices about what and how much to eat, and how much to exercise —which can be as simple as adding a thirty-minute walk to your day and a little resistance or weight training to your exercise routine.

Glucose Metabolism

When we eat a bowl of oatmeal for breakfast with a few almonds and dried cranberries and a little milk on top, our stomach starts to break down the food into components it can use. The almonds and milk are converted to amino acids (protein) and fat. The carbohydrates from the oatmeal, cranberries, and lactose in the milk are broken down into sugars (glucose). Then, a signal flies to the pancreas that there's been a load of sugar that needs to be delivered to the cells within the brain, muscles, and every other part of the body for the energy and fuel that keeps us going. The pancreas responds to this signal by releasing a pulse of insulin.

Insulin is like the outgoing friend who always brings a nice yummy tray of cupcakes (in this case, energy in the form of sugar) to a party. Insulin knows everybody, makes the rounds, and can always get into the best parties, because it's bringing the cupcakes (energy), and after all, who doesn't love cupcakes. The cells are receptive to insulin's knock at the door, with the promise of a big rush of energy in the form of sugar. Sure, come on in, we love energy! And thus insulin plus the party tray of sugar gets whisked in the cells to deliver the energy.

Insulin Resistance

If we keep asking our pancreas to pump out large amounts of insulin, let's say after eating two baskets of tortilla chips with a frozen strawberry margarita, a burrito with rice and beans, followed by a chocolate lava cake, which all gets converted into sugar, then eventually the pancreas and our cells get a little snarky. Like your favorite Real Housewife, they get tired and become a bit passive-aggressive. They're kind of fed up with way too much sugar deliveries too often and decide not to be as receptive to insulin's knock at the door. The cells don't open the door as quickly or as wide as they used to because they're full. They become: resistant to insulin.

The pancreas, frankly, is also tired of partying. It can't keep up with the huge deliveries of sugar that have been repeated for years and years. What happens is that with less insulin available to deliver the sugar and fewer cells interested in receiving the delivery, the blood sugar levels rise higher and higher and higher. A lot of the excess blood sugar gets converted into fat, and over time, chronically high blood sugar levels lead to diabetes. Diabetes also leads to more fat and more risk for heart disease.

As the amount of fat increases at the waist, our cells become even more resistant to insulin and this raises blood sugar levels, increasing the conversion of glucose to fatty acids and triglycerides, which leads to elevations in LDL cholesterol (the "bad" cholesterol) and more fat deposition. It's a vicious cycle.

Meanwhile, Back at the Liver

At the same time that insulin is delivering glucose to the cells, a little glucose goes to the liver to be converted into glycogen, which is a ready source of energy that helps maintain our blood glucose levels even when we haven't eaten, like when we're sleeping. This is important because we always need some extra stores of glycogen that can readily make a little glucose when needed as energy for our brains and body to function. Our bodies have to have readily available energy to run away from lions, to run to a meeting, or to just get out of bed in the morning.

And yet, the liver can only store so much glycogen. When there's no more room at the inn, so to speak, the extra glucose not needed for fuel and not needed for glycogen storage will be converted to another ready energy source, triglycerides. Triglycerides are fatty acids made from, you guessed it, glucose! Imagine that? A bowl of oatmeal can and often does turn into fat. Really, you don't have to eat fat to make fat.

Where does that extra fat go? Well, as you probably guessed, it goes all over your body, to the upper arms, the chin, the hips, and to your menopausal body's new favorite location, your midsection, thank you very little!

In addition, that extra glucose that was converted to triglycerides has another function. Triglycerides are not only a great source of energy but the main building block for LDL cholesterol (low density lipoprotein cholesterol), which is the type of cholesterol that can lead to heart disease. Triglycerides in small amounts are essential for health, but in large quantities they are not our friends.

How Women Lose Weight Versus How Men Do It

Have you ever noticed that men lose weight differently than women? I joke that a man can stop thinking about food (and beer) and drop ten pounds, while a woman has to run a marathon every day and eat nothing but celery and cucumbers for two weeks to lose an ounce. If she even glances at a cookie, then four pounds is immediately deposited onto her hips faster than you can say "Hold the whipped cream on the mocha, please." Eating a cookie? Forget about it! Ten pounds minimum arrives at light speed. I'm exaggerating, but you get the idea.

It's not the same for men. The truth is that men have a lot more lean muscle mass. Their muscles are like furnaces that need to be fed a steady diet of fuel. Although most women would disagree, men are always multitasking when it comes to metabolism. Men can burn 3,000 calories just by reaching for a bag of chips from their seat on the couch while watching the Patriots play the Cowboys. Then when they get up to grab a beer, they're burning 50,000 calories. Again, I exaggerate, but that couch potato in your living room is maddeningly more efficient at losing weight than you are. That is, unless you rip a page out of their playbook. I don't mean sit on the couch watching sports. I mean it's time to build up more lean muscle mass.

And yes, I know that there are also many men who have a lot of weight to lose. I'm just lamenting the fact that it's 10,000 times easier for them. The simple fact is that women hold on to weight longer than men do. Biologically, our bodies have to be prepared to nurture the next generation no matter how scarce food is.

You can see this played out if you watch *Survivor*. The men, no matter what their size, lose weight much more rapidly than the women. And if you've noticed, the women on the show who are carrying more weight also lose weight much more slowly than the overweight men on the show.

If we haven't eaten in a while, our bodies will first go to the liver and request that the glycogen stored there be released for fuel. When the glycogen stores are depleted, then our bodies ask that the fat that was stored from excess glucose be reconverted back to energy. This is how reducing calorie intake and increasing calorie output from exercise ultimately helps us lose weight and fat. But this is just part of the weight-loss equation.

Restrictive Diets and Ghrelin

We've all heard of diets that have you eat just one thing for two weeks. The lemon juice diet, the tomato diet, the bacon diet. I'm making these up, but you get the idea of very restrictive diets that have people eat 500 to 800 calories a day. Just about everyone can stay on a restrictive diet for two weeks, and they will usually see a three- to five-pound weight loss. What are they really losing? On a restrictive diet, the body will humor us and release a little excess water. Most people will notice that they're urinating more frequently at the start of a diet and that their clothes may not seem so tight. *Wow,* they think, *I'm really losing fat this time. I'm going to get into those skinny jeans for sure.* However, though they may be losing some fat, they're also losing water and also losing what they want to retain, their lean muscle mass. The loss of muscle mass will make it harder in the long run to burn calories, maintain the weight loss once they stop, and lose more weight after they get tired of eating the same tiny portions of whatever it is for more than two weeks.

The other thing that happens when most women diet is that two hormones, leptin and ghrelin, exert their influence. Leptin is the hormone that helps regulate energy expenditure and metabolism. Ghrelin helps regulate appetite and how much food we eat. When our hunter-gatherer ancestors were faced with a famine and shortage of food, it was the job of leptin to make certain that women slowed down their metabolism enough to retain enough fat to be able to carry a pregnancy to term even when there was a shortage of food. Leptin was an adaptive response to the threat of starvation.

Ghrelin is the culprit behind what many of us refer to as the "buffet binging" phenomenon. Ghrelin and other neurochemicals urge us to eat whenever we see food in front of us. No matter how abundant the food supply is, or how many times we've had the experience that there will actually be another meal available in about four hours, our brains are hardwired by ghrelin to eat and consume every single food in front of us. Ghrelin is the tiny voice in your head that says, "Eat the brownie!" And as more fat accumulates in our midsection, more ghrelin is produced, leading many women to feel as if they're hungry all the time. It's a vicious cycle. But don't despair. It can be overcome without wiring your jaw shut or running a marathon every day.

The See Food Diet Phenomena

It's called the See Food Diet, because when you see food, you eat it. Blame ghrelin. It's why being presented with a small plate of food with reasonably sized portions helps people eat less than allowing them to serve themselves and fill up their supersized plates from an abundant platter.

You have to have a pretty sophisticated cerebral cortex in your brain to override those instinctual urges to eat the cheesecake, because your brain is shouting at you, "You better have that cheesecake right now—don't delay. This might be your only chance ever to taste this. Hurry up and eat it, because you may never see a cheesecake like this again, and by the way, there could be a famine and no cheesecakes ever again starting tomorrow."

Even though you know for certain that you're going to have a gazillion more opportunities to have cheesecake, your brain is creating just enough doubt that you give in. "Well, just this once," you say, apologizing to your cerebral cortex, who shrugs because it knows that there are very powerful instincts working against you here.

The next time you're at a party or conference where there's a buffet, stand back and watch the crush of people stampeding toward the tables, no matter the quality of the food. I've often found myself thinking, *It looks like these people have never seen food before.* And in a sense, their brains, under the influence of ghrelin, are shouting, "You might never see this again, better fill up now, because you just never know if there will be a famine tomorrow." The cerebral cortex barely has a chance to hold you back from joining the line, grabbing a plate the size of Kentucky, and filling it up. I've seen this happen at medical conferences where healthcare providers line up, jostle for a place in line, and load up their plates with enough food to feed an entire town. It's difficult to resist, even for people who presumably know a lot about nutrition.

There's another aspect to the buffet-binging phenomenon that bears mentioning. That aspect is whether there is a direct monetary cost that must be paid. If a buffet is part of a wedding, a party, included in your room rate, and the cost is hidden or already paid for, then the stampede is different than if you had to pony up cash for a plateful of food. When the cost has already been covered or is hidden, then people go absolutely nuts. "All this food and it's free! Holy cow!" your instincts scream. "What are you waiting for, you idiot? Get in line before it's all gone."

Why We Put the Weight Right Back On After Dieting

Back to *Survivor*. You've seen what happens to the contestants after they come off the island. They put the weight back on. That's what happens with a lot of us, too. It's hard to keep the weight off because of our old friends leptin and ghrelin. After a restrictive diet, leptin works to slow down our metabolism and ghrelin works to increase appetite. These two hormones are part of a delicate balance that leads to gaining back all or most of the weight we lost and then a little extra just in case we encounter another famine.

Our bodies have evolved to store energy in the form of fat for the lean times. The problem is that in our modern, daily lives, there really aren't any lean times. We have an overabundance of food available to us 24/7.

Why the Scale Doesn't Budge

Chris was discouraged when she didn't see the scale move or the pounds magically disappear after weeks of working out. I've counseled many patients like Chris that our bodies will ignore our exercise and restricted calories until they see that we really mean business—that there *isn't a* famine, and we *can* eat enough food to justify revving up our metabolism from regular exercise. What's happening below the surface isn't apparent on the scale immediately. It takes time for the exercise to use up the stored glycogen and start using fat for fuel, and remember, there's less muscle mass to burn the calories. So unless you're building muscle while losing fat, you won't see any difference for a while. It will be a slow process, which can be discouraging, especially if you're on a restrictive diet and feeling deprived.

HOW TO LOSE WEIGHT: THE REAL SECRET

Losing weight around menopause requires a combination of three things. Ready for the secrets?

First, eliminate emotional eating by increasing your awareness of what and why you eat. Second, build up more lean muscle mass with resistance and weight training. Third, eat smaller portions of food regularly throughout the day for fuel and reduce your carbohydrate intake.

Really, that's all it takes. Reduce excess blood sugar. Increase the ability to burn calories by increasing muscle mass, and finally, be more mindful of every choice with food and drink. Okay, now that you know that, I'll give you some more tips on how to integrate this knowledge into your life.

The trick is to figure out how to have your favorite foods, enjoy and savor them, and decide if the taste and the amount you consumed satisfied your physical hunger and also whatever emotional attachment you have to the food, drink, or experience.

It's important to have a balanced approach, not to look at weight loss as all or nothing and to avoid deprivation. There will always be some foods that are so delicious that you absolutely must have them, and it would be wrong and also counterproductive to eliminate them from your diet completely, forever and ever. Notice I said some foods, not all foods, because of course, there are many people with food allergies or conditions that require some food restrictions. But if you have no food restrictions, then you will be able to find ways to work in the foods you love.

Increasing Awareness

One of the best ways to lose the meno potbelly and keep it off is to increase your awareness of what you're eating and why you're choosing to eat it. It's estimated that we each make between 100 and 300 decisions about food every day. Deconstructing some of the choices we make about what to eat and how much to eat, and being more mindful is the first step in developing more awareness about our relationship with food.

Choosing to pick up the fork and have the cheesecake seems like one simple choice, but really there's a lot behind it. Yes, it looks good, and it's going to taste good, but are you hungry for more than just food? Is the cheesecake filling you up physically and emotionally? Does cheesecake remind you of a special occasion? Do you feel that you need a treat right now? Are you bored? What else is going on right now that makes cheesecake or even a slice of cheese the answer?

I ask my patients who want to get to a healthier weight to keep a food diary (see the Sample Food Diary on the opposite page). I ask them to develop more awareness by writing down what they're eating and what else is going on when they're making food choices. Are they hungry? Stressed? Tired? Is the food compensating for something that's missing? Has it been a hard day and a treat would make life a bit more enjoyable?

I am inviting you to look back on the last twenty-four hours and ask yourself what you ate and what was going on when you made the choices you made. Were you physically hungry? Did you eat just enough or a bit too much? Did it taste so great, you wanted more? Could you have been physically satisfied with half or one-third the amount?

Try this for a few days to be more conscious about the motivations and feelings that surround food choices. What's really behind the impulse to pick up a latte before work or on the way to a meeting? Are you anxious and want to have a cup of comfort first? Is it a mindless routine? Would a glass of water be just as physically satisfying, but not satisfy the other needs?

This is just something to start thinking about and become more aware of. Eventually, as you notice the decisions that swirl around food and drink choices, you'll become more aware of what is happening before you make the choice and may be able to make healthier choices. Once a person starts making conscious decisions about food and weighs the benefits of healthy eating and better overall health, their weight loss becomes more sustainable.

SAMPLE FOOD DIARY

Breakfast

Coffee with 1 teaspoon sugar and 1 tablespoon Half & Half

1 egg scrambled with 1 ounce low-fat cheese

$1/2$ slice high-protein, low-carb bread

Salsa

Midmorning Snack

Low-fat string cheese with 12 roasted almonds (wanted to have chocolate after getting an upsetting email)

Lunch (out with friend)

Mixed green salad with grilled salmon, dressing on the side

Water

Midafternoon Snack

Tangerine

$1/4$ cup hummus with carrots, celery, and cherry tomatoes

Vegetable juice

Dinner

Roasted chicken, skin removed

1 cup sautéed broccoli

$1/2$ cup rice

Mixed salad

Water

Snack

Cup of hot peppermint tea

Sliced apples with 1 tablespoon peanut butter

Exercise: Walked the dog for forty-five minutes.

Emotional Triggers: Emails in the morning made me want to reach for chocolate chips; took the dog for a walk and munched on almonds instead. Lunch with friend: wanted a burger, but decided ahead of time to have a salad.

MY FOOD DIARY

Breakfast

Midmorning Snack

Lunch

Midafternoon Snack

Dinner

Evening Snack

Exercise:

Emotional Triggers:

Getting Exercise

Chris was wondering why she couldn't seem to lose her meno potbelly despite training for a mini-triathlon. What I guessed is that because she didn't exercise daily—but instead saved up all her exercise for the weekends—she didn't burn fat calories as efficiently as she could have. Her body just wasn't about to release all its stored energy during occasional exercise, even if it was intense.

I'm also certain that Chris had difficulty because she had lost lean muscle mass. It's difficult to build up lean muscle mass from just aerobic activity. What's necessary is to use weights and resistance training when working out to induce the proliferation of lean muscle mass. Even a small increase in lean muscle mass will pay big dividends in the amount of calories that are burned.

Yes, it means either getting some weights to use at home, learning how to use the machines at the gym, or finding other ways to build muscle mass from using medicine balls, barbells, or taking a class that incorporates weights or resistance into a cardio workout.

Aim for weight training at least three times each week for one-half hour. Start with weights that you're completely comfortable lifting, even if you're only lifting the bar with no weight attached. Within weeks you'll be able to lift more weight and will feel stronger. Soon you'll notice that you're more toned and that your clothes are starting to loosen. Your thigh muscles, the quadriceps, are the largest muscles in your body and a good place to start replacing fat with more muscle fibers. Leg presses are easy for most women, as it only involves sitting on a slight incline with legs extended and feet on a large flat panel that is pushed in and out slowly.

With any weight or resistance training, be sure that your body is positioned correctly, because you don't want to strain your back or neck trying to use weights from an awkward position. Take it slowly and don't attempt to lift any weight that's too heavy as this could cause a serious injury. Do take advantage of the trainers and gym staff for advice and guidance.

Women's health and exercise magazines are also a great source of weight and resistance training ideas that you can do at home with rubber bands, medicine balls, and other in-home equipment. The key is to find what works for you and incorporate it into your routine, even if it means holding onto gallon jugs of water as you do biceps curls. If you have limited time or limited access to a gym, try wearing $^1/_2$- to 2-pound ankle weights during the day to strengthen and build muscles while toning the legs.

Reducing Carbs

As it turns out, not all carbs are created equal. Food is food is food and calories from carbs are just calories right? Well, yes and no. Just as two-buck Chuck red wine from Trader Joe's is red wine, it's a little different from the 2007 Cabernet from Silver Oak. They're both red wine, but they are different. And while a nice head of iceberg lettuce is lettuce and has the same calorie count as a head of dark red leaf lettuce, the amount of water and nutrients bite for bite are also quite different.

When we look at what we eat, we also have to pay attention to how our bodies use the calories and nutrients from carbohydrates for fuel or for storage. It really doesn't matter what terms are used to help us remember that some carbs are more likely to lead to fat deposits and some are more likely to be used quickly for energy with very little left over to be converted into fat.

High-Carb Foods

- Beans (including green beans)
- Bread
- Candy
- Cereals
- Cookies
- Corn
- Crackers
- Flour-containing foods
- Fruit
- Fruit Juice
- Grains (i.e., oatmeal, quinoa, barley)
- Honey
- Pasta
- Peas
- Potatoes
- Rice
- Sweets
- Sugar-containing foods (i.e., jams, jellies, maple syrup)
- Tortillas

Some other foods also contain a few carbohydrates:
- Milk—lactose milk sugar
- Most vegetables contain a negligible amount of carbs

You've heard various terms around carbs: good carbs, bad carbs, sugar busters, the glycemic index, simple or complex carbs, absolute number of carbs, the net carbs, or the insoluble fiber content in carbs. In my mind, it really doesn't matter what you call it, as long as it works for you. The key is to figure out for yourself whether eating a particular food will deliver so much added glucose that some of it will be converted to fat and then deciding if it's worth it.

The goal is to understand that all carbs are not created or metabolized equally. We all know that fruit is not only delicious and naturally sweet but that it's also part of a healthy diet. However, there are big differences in the amount of carbohydrate that's converted to sugar and the amount of pectin (fiber in fruit) in the fruit. So knowing a bit more about the carbohydrate count in different foods will give you the tools to make healthier choices. Knowing that a glass of orange juice has almost twice as many carbs as an orange can help you make the decisions about what to eat. It's easier for me to think in terms of grams of net carbs—that is, the amount of carbs left after subtracting the fiber. The tables below can help:

TABLE 11.1. CARBOHYDRATE COUNT OF VARIOUS FOODS

FRUITS	TOTAL CARBS	FIBER	NET CARBS
Apple	19 g	3 g	16 g
Apple Juice (8 fl oz.)	29 g	0 g	29 g
Apricot	4 g	1 g	3 g
Dried Apricots (6 halves)	13 g	2 g	11 g
Apricot Juice (8 fl oz.)	33 g	1 g	32 g
Banana	31 g	4 g	27 g
1/2 cup Blueberries	28 g	2 g	26 g
Peach	15 g	2 g	13 g
1/2 cup Strawberries	6 g	2 g	4 g
Orange	15 g	3 g	12 g
Orange Juice	23 g	1 g	22 g

GRAINS & BEANS	TOTAL CARBS	FIBER	NET CARBS
1 slice of white bread	13 g	1 g	12 g
1 slice of wheat bread	12 g	1 g	11 g
1 slice of CA style protein bread	15 g	2 g	13 g
1 medium-sized flour tortilla	15 g	1 g	14 g
1 small corn tortilla	11 g	2 g	9 g
1 whole-wheat reduced-carb tortilla	10 g	7 g	3 g
1/2 cup oatmeal	14 g	2 g	12 g
1/2 cup boxed cereal (average)	16 g	4 g	12 g
1/2 cup cooked pasta	20 g	1 g	19 g
1/2 cup cooked rice (white)	22 g	0 g	22 g
1/2 cup refried beans	24 g	7 g	17 g
1/2 cup baked beans	27 g	7 g	20 g
1/2 cup green string beans (raw)	4 g	2 g	2 g
1/2 cup peas	13 g	4 g	9 g
1 baked white potato	34 g	3 g	31 g
1 baked sweet potato	41 g	6 g	35 g
1 cup French fries	48 g	4	44 g
1 ear corn on the cob	14 g	2 g	12 g
12 tortilla chips	18 g	2 g	16 g
VEGETABLES			
1 cup raw spinach	1 g	1 g	0 g
1/2 cup creamed spinach	9 g	1 g	8 g
1 cup steamed broccoli	8 g	5 g	3 g
1 cup lettuce	1 g	1 g	0 g

VEGETABLES (CONT.)	TOTAL CARBS	FIBER	NET CARBS
1/2 cup baby carrots	6 g	2 g	4 g
2 stalks celery	4 g	2 g	2 g
1/2 cup cherry tomatoes	3 g	1 g	2 g
1/2 cup sliced cucumber	1 g	0 g	1 g
1/2 cup raw peppers	4 g	1 g	3 g
6 spears asparagus	4 g	2 g	2 g
NUTS			
1/4 cup peanuts (handful ~40)	6 g	2 g	4 g
1 tablespoon peanut butter	3 g	1 g	2 g
1/4 cup almonds	8 g	4 g	4 g
1/4 cup walnuts	4 g	2 g	2 g
1/4 cup pecans	4 g	3 g	1 g
DAIRY			
1 cup fat-free milk	12 g	0 g	12 g
1 cup whole milk	11 g	0 g	11 g
1 cup nonfat Greek yogurt	9 g	0 g	9 g
1 cup low-fat fruit-flavored yogurt sweetened with sugar	46 g	0 g	46 g
1/2 cup cottage cheese	4 g	0 g	4 g
1/2 cup ricotta cheese	4 g	0 g	4 g
1 slice cheddar cheese	1 g	0 g	1 g
1 low-fat string cheese	3 g	0 g	3 g
1 wedge of Laughing Cow® cheese	1 g	0 g	1 g
1 small wedge of brie (3 oz.)	0 g	0 g	0 g

What you can see from the tables is that eating a banana and eating a bowl of strawberries both can satisfy your sweet tooth, but one will provide five times as many carbs. You may have also noticed that when fruit is juiced there's more carbohydrate, and likewise when it's dried, the sugars are more concentrated. Juicing removes the fiber that fills you up, helps prevent constipation, and helps prevent an overload of sugar all at once.

It's the same principle behind eating an ear of corn or eating a bag of corn chips. The processing removes most of the fiber, concentrates the carbs into a smaller bite-sized package, and has the net result of delivering a huge glucose load.

The goal is to eat more complex carbohydrates that have lots of fiber. For example:

- Corn tortillas instead of flour tortillas

- Brown rice instead of white rice

- Beans instead of mashed potatoes

- One-half cup of strawberries instead of a slice of banana bread

Read the Labels and Add Up the Carbs

The next step when deciding what to eat is to read the labels on packaged foods, like yogurt, salad dressing, canned soups, or anything that comes in a box or container. Trying to lose weight? You reach for the yogurt, and then look at the label. If it's got fruit or flavoring, even if it's low fat, it may have 30 or more grams of carbohydrate in it. If it's plain nonfat, it may have less than 5 grams.

Here's the net carbs in the Mexican meal:

2 baskets of chips	32 g
1 frozen strawberry margarita	17 g
1 burrito	35 g
$1/2$ cup of beans	17 g
$1/2$ cup rice	24 g
1 small chocolate lava cake	62 g
Total:	**A whopping: 187 g**

How about breakfast: Oatmeal, dried cranberries, almonds, and a few drops of milk?

Sugar in your coffee? Cha-ching, it adds up quickly.

Sandwich or salad at lunch? Pizza for dinner. Thin crust or thicker crust?

A few slices of bread while waiting for your entrée?

French fries instead of salad?

It all adds up.

* *

Nurse Barb's Smart Tips to Reduce Carbs

Stay within this suggested number of grams of carbs each day based on your height:

5'0"–5'3"	100–140	5'9"–6'0"	160–180
5'3"–5'6"	120–160	6'0" and over	180–200
5'6"–5'9"	140–180		

* *

Nurse Barb's Sexy Sample Menu with Carb Count

Breakfast

1 egg with low-fat cheese = 1 g

1 slice of high-protein bread = 9 g

Water, coffee, or tea with calorie-free sweetener = 0 g

Snack

Low-fat string cheese = 3 g

12 almonds = 2 g

Tomato or vegetable juice = 6 g

Lunch

Salad with fat-free balsamic vinaigrette, peppers, tomato, and carrots (hold the carbs, including croutons, beans, corn, tortilla chips) = 8 g

Chicken breast or salmon = 0 g

1 cup of skim milk or fat-free plain Greek yogurt mixed with $1/2$ cup strawberries or blueberries = 10g

Water = 0 g

Snack

Celery and $1/2$ cup low-fat cottage cheese = 5 g

$1/2$ orange = 6 g

Dinner

Salmon filet = 0 g

Salad = 5 g

Vegetable (1 cup broccoli) = 3 g

1 square of dark chocolate = 13 g

TOTAL = 71 g Net Carbs

Nurse Barb's Sexy Sample Menu 2 with Carb Count

Breakfast

2 slices of turkey rolled around softened low-fat cheese = 1 g

Water, coffee, tea with sugar-free sweetener if preferred = 1 g

Snack

$1/2$ cup low-fat cottage cheese mixed with blueberries = 10 g

Lunch

Open-faced burger made with high-protein, low-carb bread and topped with lettuce, tomato, onion, avocado, pickles, cheese = 12 g

Side salad = 6 g

Unsweetened tea or water = 0 g

Snack

$\frac{1}{2}$ cup Greek yogurt or low-fat ricotta cheese mixed with a handful of walnuts, almonds, or pecans = 6 g

1 cup of tomato or other vegetable juice = 6 g

Dinner

Roasted chicken (breast or thigh), 2 small pieces = 0 g

Roasted carrots, onions, and peppers (1 cup) = 18 g

Sautéed spinach or chard with garlic = 2 g

$\frac{1}{2}$ cup creamy polenta = 24 g

2 small apricots, plums, or a peach = 10 g

TOTAL = 96 g Net Carbs

For more menu plans and recipes, visit www.NurseBarb.com.

YOU CAN LOSE THE MENO POTBELLY!

It's never too late to get healthier. Losing the meno potbelly will not only help you look and feel better, with less belly fat, you'll be at less risk of diabetes and heart disease. It's not going to happen overnight, but with more mindful choices, fewer carbs, and more weight training you can absolutely be trimmer, leaner, and stronger, and yes, a lot sexier!

Think about all of the choices you make around food and drink. You'll be amazed at what you're thinking and feeling when you open the fridge looking for answers or find yourself eating something just because it's there. Listening to hunger cues and then deciding how to fill that void is another important step in the process.

At first, looking at the amount of carbohydrates in food may seem a bit over the top and obsessive, but in time, most people alter their eating and shopping habits. In the past, the lure of the middle section of the grocery store may have been too much to resist, but after reading labels, many people start buying from the produce, meat, dairy, and cheese sections and cooking healthier choices. Moving toward a diet that's vegetable dominant with less high-fat protein and fewer carbs is not only a great way to get the skinny jeans on without lying down to zip them up, but it will help you feel better and have more energy. As you lose weight, your confidence will soar as will the sexiness quotient.

And finally, exercise is essential for all of us. If you're already exercising, you know how much better you feel. Adding weights to your workout will make all the difference in adding lean muscle mass, which is essential around menopause. The more muscle you have, the faster you'll burn calories and see the meno potbelly shrink. But there are so many more benefits. You may be surprised to learn that just thirty minutes of regular exercise each day is associated with a decreased risk of breast and other cancers. Being stronger means you can do more of the things you enjoy, whether it's skiing or cycling, hiking or dancing, gardening, or traveling; it's all easier when you have the strength and stamina.

13

Plugging the "Leak"

*H*ow many times have you suffered in silence, concentrating fiercely on holding off the overpowering urge to run to the bathroom? Do you know where every clean bathroom is in a five-mile radius of your house? Do you plan shopping excursions based on which department stores have decent bathrooms? Do you limit the amount of liquids you drink after 7 PM, so that you have a decent chance of sleeping a few hours before popping up like a Ping-Pong ball all night to visit the bathroom? Do you wear panty liners or thicker protection every day for the little and big leaks that are inevitable? If you answered yes to any of these questions, you're not alone. You're in the same leaky boat as half of women over fifty. Half! That's right, 50 percent of us deal with some type of leaky bladders.

Many women are understandably hesitant to discuss this issue with anyone, not even their girlfriends. Leaking is the ultimate taboo topic in menopause. Compounding this problem is the hesitancy many healthcare providers have in bringing up incontinence and leaking with their patients. Study after study shows that most women will not bring up this sensitive issue because they feel uncomfortable, they sense discomfort in their providers, and they don't think there are any decent treatment options. Many women would rather talk about their weight than talk about leaking urine. And we all know how uncomfortable it is to talk about weight.

It's virtually impossible to feel hot and sexy and in the mood for love when there's even the slightest suggestion of a hint of urine. Who wants to peel off clothes and worry about a pad with any telltale evidence? No one!

Many women are mortified by the stigma that comes with leaking urine and soiling underwear and clothes. Instead of talking about it, they do their best to adapt and go out and buy more pads. It's completely understandable that women at any age, especially at menopause, would be hesitant to ask for help with incontinence. I believe that once a woman hears herself saying, "I leak urine," suddenly the issue becomes real, altering her self-image from a healthy vibrant woman to someone who might need to wear diapers.

This is an issue that's shrouded in minipads, toilet paper, and shame. But it doesn't have to be. Having a cool sexy menopause is within every-one's reach even if there's a little or a lot of leaking. I've cared for and talked with many women who have ditched the minipads. They can run, dance, and even jump on a trampoline without leaking. They were surprised that they could get back to living their lives, without having the constant worry about their bladder betraying them. There's a solution for every woman, whether it's exercises, medications, or minimally invasive surgery.

Leaking urine is another taboo topic we rarely discuss with even our closest friends. Instead, women make jokes or mention that they laughed so hard they worried about wetting their pants. The truth is many women, like Randi, Helen, Maya, and Nan, who share their stories below, are dealing with leaking urine and don't know what to do to fix it. Yet effective help for getting and staying dry is available.

RANDI'S STORY

Randi hoped no one would notice her frozen smile. "If I just sit still and not think about it, I can hold out another five minutes until everyone starts clapping," she reasoned through clenched teeth. Randi was kicking herself for not sitting closer to the exit and for not stopping off in the bathroom before the luncheon started. She couldn't concentrate on what was surely a wonderfully inspirational talk; all she could think about was getting to the ladies' room before she burst.

Randi couldn't just jump up and run for the exit, and not because of what people might think—she was well beyond that. It was her bladder, her new and unforgiving boss. Her bladder didn't allow her to jump up and down, sneeze, or even step off a curb. She had learned the hard way that when her bladder wasn't happy, she wasn't happy, and so in addition to trying to hold her urine, she also berated herself for not doing more Kegel exercises (see page 236). She vowed to start doing them this afternoon on the ride home. The trouble was, she wasn't sure if she was doing them correctly. She wasn't confident that anything except using more pads would help her situation.

Randi came in to see me, not to talk about her bladder issue, but because she thought she had the flu. She'd been sneezing and coughing throughout the day and night and had itchy, watery eyes. I was pretty sure her symptoms were related to seasonal allergies. Then, because so many health issues are interrelated, I took the opportunity to ask about leaking. "Some women leak urine when they cough or sneeze. Have you ever experienced that?" I asked. Randi hesitated, "How did you know? I just thought it was normal. I've been using a lot of pads and putting up with it."

Randi couldn't hold her urine when coughing, sneezing, or laughing; this suggested a diagnosis of stress incontinence. I explained that it wasn't the stress of worrying, it was the stress of added pressure on her bladder. Her exam revealed a significant cystocele (bladder prolapse) and her muscle tone was only a weak shadow of its former self.

After showing her a diagram of where her bladder used to be and where it was now, I showed her how to urinate twice on each visit to the bathroom, a technique known as double voiding. Randi could stand up after emptying her bladder, rock her pelvis back and forth like Elvis, and then sit back down and empty her bladder again. She was surprised that more urine was released on her second attempt. This decreased her need to go as frequently. I also asked her to begin pelvic floor physical therapy and referred her to a urogynecologist to discuss surgical options.

Randi went to the physical therapist every week for two months. She bought an electrical stimulator, which helped her improve her muscle tone. Before she knew it, her number of accidents diminished, she wasn't soaking as many pads, and her Kegels had become strong enough to keep her dry even with a sneeze. She was considering surgery but felt that it could wait a while.

HELEN'S STORY

Helen was a dignified and trusted financial executive keeping a big secret. With a Blackberry in one hand and a roll-aboard suitcase in the other, she boarded a six-hour flight. Although she could have used a drink to unwind, she had decided not to drink anymore on flights, because that meant more trips to the tiny airplane bathrooms.

Helen made a quick preventive trip to the plane's bathroom before takeoff, knowing that she had at least two hours before needing to go again. For the last year, it seemed that no matter how much she drank, she had the urge to urinate every one and a half to two hours. Frequent trips to the bathroom through the night meant she hadn't had a good night's sleep in ages. She felt that she had to go constantly, even if there were only a few drops. Helen had resorted to wearing thick pads to soak up the dribbles and the accidents that were becoming more and more common. The worst part was the unrelenting feeling that she had to go, again and again and again.

Everything would have been just fine on this trip, if it hadn't been for the %^@* turbulence. Helen wasn't concerned about her bladder yet; she knew from experience that she had about thirty minutes before she would have some turbulence of her own. She focused on the spreadsheet on her laptop; however, twenty minutes later, Helen's insistent urge to urinate became much stronger than the plane's rocky ride. She knew she was headed for big trouble if she didn't get to the bathroom right this minute. Helen weighed the alternatives. She was wearing a pad, but would it be enough? Could she get to the bathroom without being scolded by the flight attendants? Did she really care if they scolded her? Would she have an accident? How much longer could this turbulence last? How much longer could she last?

These are the kinds of dilemmas that no one should ever have to deal with, especially at 36,000 feet. After six of the longest minutes of her life, Helen made an executive decision, unbuckled her seat belt, and without a glance back, quickly slipped into the bathroom and locked the door. Okay, I'm safe, she thought. But unfortunately, she wasn't safe. Suddenly, just as she was turning around to put the seat down, her worst fears came true.

She was too late. Her bladder punished her for waiting and opened the floodgates. Her thick pad was quickly overwhelmed.

Helen called me when she landed. I asked her to keep a bladder diary (see Evaluation, later in this chapter) for a few days and make an appointment. When she came in for her appointment, her diary, her symptoms of having the urge to urinate frequently throughout the day and night, combined with her leaking a large amount during her flight, all added up to a diagnosis of an overactive bladder (OAB). In this condition, the bladder sends an insistent and uncomfortable urge to go, go, go, or in a cruel twist, it may take matters into its own hands and forcefully expel larger quantities of urine, not just little drips or leaks.

Helen was thirty pounds over a healthy weight. Her physical exam and lab tests confirmed that the extra weight put her into the prediabetic category. I wondered if that might be contributing to some mild nerve damage that would worsen OAB. She was free of bladder and vaginal infections, though her vagina was dry, which also contributes to this condition (see Chapter 8).

After reviewing her bladder diary, I outlined a variety of treatment options starting with a weight-loss plan. I suggested a bladder relaxation and retraining plan. First, she needed to relearn how to ignore the strong, insistent urges her bladder was sending without leaking, and use a pelvic floor physical therapy class to maximize the benefits of her Kegel exercises (see page 236). Then I asked Helen to schedule urination every two hours, avoid caffeine in the afternoons, and limit her liquid intake after 6 PM I saw Helen a few weeks later, and although she reported some improvement with the diet restriction and the bladder retraining, it still wasn't enough.

She was ready to consider a prescription medication. These work to help decrease bladder contractions, which send the insistent signals that it's time to urinate. There are oral tablets, a twice-weekly patch, and a gel that all produce a 60 to 75 percent improvement in symptoms. Helen was ready to stop her nighttime ritual of three visits to the bathroom and start sleeping more. She was willing to put up with the side effects of the medication, which include dry mouth, dry eyes, and constipation.

When she came back a month later, she reported that she was doing

*very well, had retrained her bladder, and was weaning herself off the med-
ication. I also discussed with Helen the option of stimulating the sacral
nerve in case her symptoms worsened in the future. Known as sacral nerve
neuromodulation or InterStim, this is an implantable device that has helped
women whose leaking hasn't responded to other treatments.*

MAYA'S STORY

*Maya was a stay-at-home mom who had plenty on her plate caring for her
family and volunteering in the schools. Maya also had another special skill.
Like a bladder-focused GPS, she knew precisely where every bathroom was
in a ten-mile radius of her house. She not only knew if there was a bathroom at each of the local soccer fields but she also knew if it was likely to
be clean. When it came to the mall, Maya knew the best place to park so
that she could make the shortest beeline to the penultimate clean ladies
lounge at Nordstrom's. Other department store restrooms were clean, but
there were too many detours through racks of clothes to get to them fast.
She also knew where the bathrooms in every grocery, coffee shop, and
pharmacy were.*

*She was on her way home from another one of the kids' practices
when she realized that she'd never make it. She silently ticked off some of
her options as she drove home. She should have used the bathroom at the
field. I could stop for some milk at Whole Foods and scoot past the fish
section, or maybe Safeway and head straight back to the dairy wall, or
CVS might be faster because it's a straight shot to the restroom by the
pharmacy, she thought. Maya sometimes felt that she could write a
Michelin-like guide to bathrooms and rate them with stars or a faucet
logo. She smiled to herself as she mused about taking the time to write a
bathroom guide.*

*Although she was wearing a substantial pad for these kinds of "just in
case" emergencies, she was still nervous about the likelihood of getting all
the way home, putting the key in the door, and then not being able to get
to the bathroom in time.*

She didn't understand why something as incongruous as putting a key in the lock of her front door would be the one thing that triggered her bladder to leak. She had never heard of anyone with this problem. Sure, she had laughed along with her friends at Bunco, who joked about peeing their pants when they laughed or sneezed. That was something she could understand from the change in pressure, but this? Jingling her keys? It didn't make sense. Luckily she had been practicing Kegel exercises after each of her children were born and could keep the flow somewhat contained, but lately it had been getting more difficult to keep her pads dry. She also felt a bulging sensation around her vagina, as if things were falling out.

Maya was relieved to know that her "key in the lock" type of incontinence, also known as urge incontinence, was common and that the bulging she felt could be corrected. She promptly began going to pelvic floor physical therapy classes, and though she saw some improvement, she was interested in a permanent fix. I referred her to a urogynecologist who suggested a sling procedure, which changed Maya's life. (See Surgical Treatments later in this chapter.) After her surgery, she could run with her kids, jump on the trampoline, and didn't have to hit every bathroom in the mall.

NAN'S STORY

Nan came to see me for vaginal itching and odor. Once in the office, she also complained of having to urinate constantly, some leaking, and a burning pain as the flow started. She was afraid that her recent leaking signaled the beginning of menopause, even though she was still having periods and only had an occasional night sweat. She wanted to be seen right away, since the itching was keeping her up at night and the pain with urination was getting worse. It wasn't like the bladder infections she had in the past, which made her more worried about what else might be going on. Nan was discouraged. She was scared that once leaking started it would become an inevitable part of her life.

After listening to her symptoms, doing an examination, and testing her urine and vaginal discharge, I was able to reassure Nan that what she was *experiencing was a combination of a bladder infection and a vaginal infection caused by bacterial vaginosis. These were very likely both the result of vaginal dryness and changes in the pH that were just beginning (see Chapter 8). I was hopeful that by treating both infections, her leaking would stop. I also gave her instructions for using vaginal estrogen to help prevent this from recurring in the future.*

Nan practically skipped in for her return visit. All of her symptoms had vanished, she happily reported, including the leaking. Was it really just a result of the bladder infection? She wanted to know more about prevention and the cause of her recent leaking.

THE NITTY-GRITTY ON URINARY PROBLEMS

Let me just say that gravity is *not* our friend when it comes to our bladders and leaking. That's right. Sir Isaac Newton can take his apple and well, you get the idea. Basically, the reason that many urinary problems occur around the time of menopause is the supporting muscles of the pelvic floor start to weaken and that's when trouble starts.

Staying Dry

In order for a woman to stay dry, she needs to have:

- Some strength in her pelvic floor muscles to counteract abdominal pressure from coughing or sneezing

- A well-functioning urethra with competent sphincters (valves) that hold back the urine

- A bladder and urethra that have support from the pelvic floor muscles

- Intact nerves that can send signals back and forth between bladder, urethra, spinal cord, and brain

- A bladder that can hold at least one-half to one cup (120 to 240 ml) of urine before pumping it out

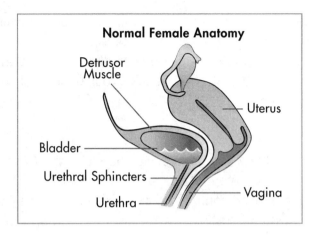

Figure 3.
Normal Female
Anatomy.

The Bladder's Healthy Nervous System

The bladder is composed of a smooth muscle, known as the detrusor, and resembles a round balloon that fills up with the urine that travels down from the kidneys through tiny tubes known as ureters (not to be confused with the urethra). The ureters bring urine to the bladder and don't typically impact leaking in the way that the urethra does. The urethra is the tube that urine travels down from the bladder to the outside of our bodies. The bladder acts much like your water heater, with the urethra acting like the faucet. The brain controls whether the faucet, in this case the urethra, is turned on or off.

The bladder has an amazing ability to stretch and expand, which holds and stores the constant stream of urine from the kidneys. As the bladder fills, the stretching of the detrusor muscles actually tells the nerves to send signals to the spinal cord that it's *not* time to go yet and to stay closed.

The spinal cord and the bladder send messages back and forth to each other, keeping the urethral sphincters (valves) closed tight and telling the bladder's muscles to stay quiet and to resist the urge to push urine out in a contraction. At the same time, those signals also alert the brain to start looking for a bathroom. Holding and releasing urine is under both voluntary (the brain's) and involuntary (the spinal cord's) control. However, there are times when it's impossible to get to the bathroom, and as long as everything is in good working order, a person's brain can override the involuntary impulses to release urine and continue to "hold" it while the bladder continues to expand. This is what happens when your bladder is full and you're driving. You can't just pull off the road to relieve yourself, so you ignore the insistent urge, holding your urine until you can find a suitable bathroom.

Involuntary Control

The bladder fills and doesn't leak without a person having to think about it. This occurs under involuntary control. The valves or sphincters in the urethra near the bladder's neck control the flow of urine by staying closed until a certain pressure is reached. If there's too much pressure, perhaps from a full bladder and the added force of a cough or sneeze, then the urethral sphincters near the bladder may open and urine may drip out.

Voluntary Control

Further down the urethra is the external sphincter, which a woman can voluntarily control using the same skeletal muscles that are squeezed with a Kegel exercise (see page 236). This voluntary squeezing closes the sphincter, preventing urine from escaping. Voluntarily relaxing opens the sphincter, enabling urine to flow.

Despite the urge to urinate, healthy people can hold their urine until they get to a bathroom. It almost seems unconscious, because for many people, just sitting on the toilet and thinking about urinating will relax the sphincter and start the flow of urine.

How Much Can the Bladder Hold?

When I was working in pediatric intensive care, there were many times I couldn't leave a patient's bedside and had to wait several hours before going to the bathroom. After an eight-hour shift drinking coffee and soda without a bathroom break, it seemed like my bladder could hold gallons of liquid.

In reality, most women's bladders can hold about two cups of fluid before the stretching sensation in the destrusor muscle signals the brain that it's time to go. The normal bladder capacity is 400 to 600 ml of fluid, or about two cups. Most people will have an "urge" to urinate at 240 ml (one cup), and many people can "hold" it for much longer. Likewise, many women are able to sleep through the night, with a full bladder holding over 500 ml (two cups) of urine, without getting up to relieve themselves.

Most bladders can hold up to 600 ml of urine (about two and a half cups) before insistent signals that it's time to go and pain sets in. Even then, the bladder can continue to stretch to hold more urine until you can go.

The kidneys make 1 ml of urine every minute.* Do the math:

- 1 hour: 2 ounces or $1/4$ cup (60 ml)

- 4 hours: 1 cup (240 ml)

- 8 hours: 2 cups (480 ml)

- 10 hours: $2^1/2$ cups (600 ml)

*More urine is made more quickly with beverages containing alcohol or caffeine.

Muscle Tone of the Pelvic Floor Muscles

The pelvic floor muscles and crisscrossing supporting ligaments in the pelvis are a sort of firm, yet flexible trampoline that cradles the uterus and bladder up nice and high, defying gravity's downward pull. The urethra and vagina pass through the pelvic floor muscles, so that when they're squeezed with a Kegel exercise (see page 236), it's similar to pulling purse strings to close off the opening. These muscles are collectively known as the *levator ani,* and include the pubococcygeal muscles. *Levator* means lifter, and that's one of the muscles' functions, to hold or lift up the pelvic organs.

We use our pelvic floor muscles every day, when we squeeze to hold urine, do a Kegel exercise, or when trying to prevent gas emissions from the rectum. Over time, with added weight, pregnancies, or loss of tone from declining estrogen levels, that trampoline, once so firm and flexible, begins to show the effects of gravity, sagging, and drooping. The crisscrossing support isn't as tight either.

Without the firm support of the pelvic floor muscles, the uterus, bladder, and urethra may also start to sag, droop, and shift their positions, interfering with normal functioning. This makes it more difficult or even impossible to squeeze the muscles and the urethra.

A prolapsed bladder is known as a cystocele. A prolapsed urethra is known as a urethracele. The uterus can also prolapse. There are varying degrees of severity that range from mild to severe with accompanying symptoms.

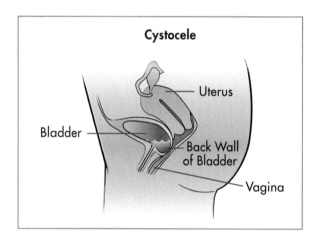

Figure 4. Cystocele from weakened pelvic floor muscles.

Prolapsed Bladder

As you can see from the illustration in Figure 4, the back wall of the bladder is drooping and has bulged downward into the vaginal space. This is a cystocele, or prolapsed bladder. As the angle of the bladder neck and urethra tilts backward, the sphincter's normal function of holding and releasing urine can be affected.

Many younger women who are a decade or two away from menopause have some degree of prolapse. Prior to menopause, many of these women are able to stay dry by compensating and squeezing their pelvic floor muscles. However, as estrogen levels decline, those once strong and powerful muscles begin to weaken, making it harder to stop urine from flowing. If the bladder and urethra shift out of place and are lower than the pelvic floor muscles, then squeezing will have little to no effect and leaking will be inevitable.

Urinary Incontinence

Millions of women deal with urinary incontinence—the accidental leak-age of urine—at some time in their lives and especially in midlife and as they get older. There are four major types of urinary incontinence and a number of treatment options available.

Stress Incontinence

When gravity exerts pressure on the bladder and urethra without the sup-port of the pelvic floor muscles providing a counterbalance, any increase in pressure over normal can stress the valves and cause leaking. Many women, like Maya, feel that there's a bulging sensation in their vagina, which represents the relaxation of the bladder wall. With the bladder out of position, leaking is more likely.

Urge Incontinence

Women have repeated and constant urges to urinate and often leak with certain triggers, such as putting a key in the lock or just glimpsing a toi-let. This occurs when a woman has had repeated experiences of having an uncomfortably full bladder and having to hold it until she can get home or get to an appropriate bathroom. Her bladder may begin to relax and leak with certain triggers, like jingling car keys, putting the key in the lock, or simply walking into the bathroom. I'm convinced that the bladder knows that relief is just seconds away from the time the key gets in the lock, and it decides it's close enough and relaxes the sphinc-ter prematurely.

Mixed Incontinence

Many women have mixed types of incontinence that are influenced by both stress and urge incontinence. The treatment is based upon the clues from a bladder diary (see page 233) and usually includes pelvic floor physical therapy, avoiding bladder irritants, and perhaps adding medica-tions that decrease trips to the bathroom. Women can expect 60 to 75 percent improvement in their symptoms, decreasing nighttime voiding, and elongating the time between trips to the bathroom with medication. What I've seen that works best is a combination of treatment options.

Overactive Bladder

Similar to urge incontinence, women have repeated and constant urges to urinate. As the bladder fills, the muscles want to squeeze urine out, despite voluntary efforts to hold it. This is what happened to Helen at 36,000 feet. Her bladder was stretching, sending urgent signals to her brain that it was time to go. By the time her bladder stretched just a little bit too much, it was too late, and the muscle revolted by pushing a large volume of urine out, overwhelming the urethral sphincters.

Leaking with a Bladder Infection

Though most leaking at midlife is chronic and not a result of a bladder infection, checking the urine for infection is an important first step. As estrogen levels start to decline with approaching menopause, sometimes the first symptoms women will notice are dryness in the vagina and more frequent urination. The vaginal and urinary tracts are particularly sensitive to small fluctuations in hormone levels. As estrogen levels start to decline, the delicate pH balance in the vagina can shift and cause our

TABLE 10.1. TYPES OF URINARY INCONTINENCE

TYPE	SYMPTOMS	CAUSES
Stress	Leakage from cough, sneeze, change in position, jumping. Leakage in small spurts or drops.	Increased abdominal pressure on bladder, with loss of support from pelvic floor muscles.
Urge	Leakage with a strong urge to urinate or with triggers such as a key in the lock, running water.	Bladder irritants. Nerve damage, overweight, infection, frequent voiding.
Mixed	Symptoms of both stress and urge incontinence.	Increases with age and all causes above.
Overactive Bladder (OAB)	Sense of urgency, frequent. May leak large volumes; nighttime visits to bathroom.	Bladder irritants. Overstretching of destrusor muscle overwhelms sphincters, causes emptying.

good and beneficial bacteria to decline, opening the window of opportunity for more harmful bacteria that cause infections to overgrow. This shift often causes a domino effect in the vagina, the urethra, and the bladder, leading to irritation, odor, and infections in both the vagina and bladder. (For more on this, see Chapter 8.)

EVALUATION AND TREATMENT FOR URINARY INCONTINENCE AND OVERACTIVE BLADDER

In order to treat leaking more effectively, it's important to have an understanding of the circumstances that influence how much urine the bladder can hold and what triggers leaking. Keeping a bladder diary that also includes the amounts and types of liquids consumed, as well as any other bladder irritants, is the first step in resolving the issue.

Bladder Diary

A bladder diary is an invaluable resource that helps us better understand the various triggers for leaking, how often it occurs, and under what circumstances, as well as the volume of urine leaked. With five to seven days of information, many practitioners can make an accurate diagnosis and recommend treatment before moving to more extensive testing with a urologist. Many women also find that keeping a bladder diary not only helps with a diagnosis but also helps them identify patterns and triggers that provoke urinating and leaking. With the added focus on the influences that wreak havoc on their bladder, they find that by simply keeping a record they're able to regain some control over the situation.

My favorite bladder diary comes from the National Institutes of Health. You can download it free of charge from their website at http://kidney.niddk.nih.gov/kudiseases/pubs/diary/diary_508.pdf.

Your Daily Bladder Diary

This diary will help you and your healthcare team figure out the causes of your bladder control trouble. The "sample" line shows you how to use the diary.

Your name: _____

Date: _____

Time	Drinks		Trips to the Bathroom		Accidental Leaks	Did you feel a strong urge to go?	What were you doing at the time?
	What kind?	How much?	How many times?	How much urine? (circle one)	How much? (circle one)	Circle one	Sneezing, exercising having sex, lifting, etc.
Sample	*Coffee*	*2 cups*	✓✓	Ⓢ ○ ○ sm med lg	○ Ⓜ ○ sm med lg	Yes (No)	*Running*
6–7 a.m.				○ ○ ○	○ ○ ○	Yes No	
7–8 a.m.				○ ○ ○	○ ○ ○	Yes No	
8–9 a.m.				○ ○ ○	○ ○ ○	Yes No	
9–10 a.m.				○ ○ ○	○ ○ ○	Yes No	
10–11 a.m.				○ ○ ○	○ ○ ○	Yes No	
11–12 noon				○ ○ ○	○ ○ ○	Yes No	
12–1 p.m.				○ ○ ○	○ ○ ○	Yes No	
1–2 p.m.				○ ○ ○	○ ○ ○	Yes No	
2–3 p.m.				○ ○ ○	○ ○ ○	Yes No	
3–4 p.m.				○ ○ ○	○ ○ ○	Yes No	
4–5 p.m				○ ○ ○	○ ○ ○	Yes No	
5–6 p.m.				○ ○ ○	○ ○ ○	Yes No	
6–7 p.m.				○ ○ ○	○ ○ ○	Yes No	

Use this sheet as a master for making copies that you can use as a bladder diary for as many days as you need.

Bladder Diary from the National Institutes of Health.

Avoid Bladder Irritants

Highly acidic foods, ones with high levels of vitamin C, and drinks with caffeine have been shown to irritate the bladder and increase the feeling of having to go "urgently." A complete list of bladder irritants includes:

- Alcohol: beer, wine, and mixed drinks
- Artificial sweeteners: all types
- Carbonated drinks
- Chocolate
- Citrus fruits and their juice: oranges, lemons, tangerines, and grapefruit
- Coffee: both caffeinated and decaf
- Colas
- Cranberries and cranberry juice
- Some fruits such as strawberries, pineapple, and guava
- Spicy foods: those made with chilies and other spices
- Sweeteners: Honey and added sugar
- Tomatoes
- Vinegar
- Vitamin C supplements

Physical Therapy for Bladder Control

Physical therapy is one of the best ways to regain control of the bladder and help minimize or stop leaking. In pelvic-floor physical therapy, a woman uses biofeedback to recognize her pelvic floor muscles and then relearns how to contract and squeeze them effectively. Physical therapy is the first step in treating all types of incontinence and overactive bladder.

Women find significant improvement after two to three classes. I have many patients who have been able to get back to running, cycling, horseback riding, and their normal lives after strengthening their muscles with pelvic-floor physical therapy.

Finding a class is as simple as asking your provider for a referral or searching online for classes in your area. You can also visit a certified physical therapist who specializes in helping women stay dry. For women who need extra help strengthening the pelvic floor, the therapist also has the option of using tiny amounts of nonpainful electrical stimulation to stimulate the muscles and help restore their function. Women may also purchase their own electrical stimulator for use in the privacy of their own home. Electrical stimulation helps muscles regain strength and control and can enhance sexual activity and pleasure with orgasms.

Pessaries

If the bladder, uterus, or pelvic floor muscles are sagging or drooping, one option is to use a pessary to push everything back up closer to where it belongs. A pessary is a flexible medical-grade rubber device that is inserted into the vagina. Similar to using a diaphragm, the pessary provides the support that pelvic floor muscles aren't able to provide. Though a few types of pessaries look like diaphragms, there are many other varieties of shapes and sizes. Pessaries have been around for many years and are good alternatives for women who aren't the best candidates for corrective surgery. Most women who use pessaries insert and remove them on their own, washing them and then reinserting. If a woman wants to have intercourse, she removes her pessary first. I have fitted patients with a pessary; they then use it for six to twelve months while contemplating surgery. I have other patients who use pessaries for many years and never have surgery.

•   •

Bladder Relaxation Plan

This plan will help reteach your bladder to expand and hold more urine without leaking.

1. As soon as there is a strong urge to urinate: do five to ten deep cleansing breaths.

2. At the same time, practice doing a Kegel exercise (see page 236) and hold it throughout the deep breaths.

3. Try to repeat this exercise five to ten times while concentrating on something completely unrelated to urinating.

4. Then after feeling calm and in control, walk slowly to the bathroom while squeezing.

5. Continue squeezing and breathing slowly while you undress and sit on the toilet.

6. When you are ready, relax to start the urine flow.

• • • • • • • • • • • • • • • • • •

Sacral Neuromodulation

For women with any symptoms of an overactive bladder, sacral neuro-modulation (SNM), known as Interstim, is a new and effective option when other treatments have failed. Essentially, a pacemaker-like device is implanted in the buttocks with a wire that extends to the nerves in the sacral area that control urine storage and emptying. Over 80 percent of patients with SNM are satisfied with how effective this option is and the control they've regained.

Medications

These work to help decrease bladder contractions, which send the insistent signals that it's time to urinate. There are oral tablets, a twice-weekly patch, and a gel that all effect between a 60 to 75 percent improvement in symptoms. With new formulations, the side effects of dry mouth, dry eyes, and constipation are being improved upon. Many women find that the benefits far outweigh any side effects.

Many providers prescribe medications for a short duration while physical therapy and other treatments are used. Women are often able to wean off the medications after they begin pelvic floor physical therapy or have surgery and regain more control over their bladders.

Surgical Treatments

If you are considering a surgical repair for leaking, the first step is to strengthen the pelvic floor muscles. This will maximize your recovery and help the tissue heal faster. It's also important to visit a urogynecologist who has extensive experience. Ask to talk to some of your surgeon's patients. Women who have the best outcomes are the ones who see specialists. There are several different surgical options available to women who have leaking:

- **SLING**—A mesh is used to pull the bladder and urethra up and support them. The ends of the sling can be attached to bone or other tissue. These procedures have evolved over the last few years and are quite effective in helping a woman regain control over her bladder.

- **VAGINAL REPAIR**—When the vaginal tissue has stretched and the pelvic floor muscles have weakened, there are a variety of surgical procedures available to correct these issues. It's best to discuss the options with a urogynecologist.

- **BURCH PROCEDURE**—Also known as a retropubic suspension, a Burch procedure helps reposition the urethra and bladder up higher in the pelvis. This procedure is rarely done now, as there are other more effective options.

Nurse Barb's Staying Dry Tips

Do Your Kegel Exercises

- If you're not sure how to do a Kegel exercise, try to squeeze your pelvic floor muscles. If you're not sure how, then think about how you'd hold your urine or try to hold back the passage of gas and squeeze, contracting those muscles.

- Notice if the muscles around your genitals and rectal area are squeezing together.

- Then, the next time your bladder is full, sit on the toilet and allow some urine to pass, then squeeze and contract those muscles and try to *HOLD* the urine or at least reduce the amount of flow. Then release and try again.

- This will help you identify those pelvic floor muscles that you'll be squeezing and contracting to do Kegel exercises.

- If you can't hold your urine or reduce the amount of flow, you'll need to have your healthcare provider or a pelvic floor physical therapist help you identify those muscles and learn how to squeeze, contract, and relax them effectively.

- Continue practicing contracting and relaxing your pelvic floor muscles for 3 seconds at a time. Relax the muscles for 3 seconds and repeat.

- Try doing sets of 10 three-second Kegels one to two times per day.

- Once you've mastered this, try holding your pelvic floor muscles with a Kegel and keeping a steady squeeze or contraction for 5 seconds, gradually working up to holding it for 10 seconds.

- Remember to breathe while contracting your pelvic floor muscles with a Kegel.

- Check the effectiveness of your Kegels by trying to stop the flow of urine and holding it for three seconds before releasing.

- Work up to doing 50 Kegels each day as this has been shown to help maintain bladder control for women well into their nineties. Really!

- Continue to practice Kegels occasionally while urinating; this is an easy way to see if your Kegels are effective.

- Link doing Kegels with activities you do several times each day, from starting your car, brushing your teeth, or checking emails.

- Practice Kegels while having intercourse. Alternating between contractions and relaxation can enhance your pleasure as well as your partner's.

Use the Double Voiding Technique

- This technique can help reduce the number of trips to the bathroom by helping to completely empty the bladder each time. The trick is to sit on the toilet and urinate, wipe or pat dry, then stand up, bend at the waist, rock forward, and then sit back down and urinate again.

- If a woman has a cystocele (prolapsed bladder), this will bring any residual urine that might be hiding in the back part of the bladder toward the front.

- You can accomplish the same thing by inserting a clean finger into the vagina after urinating and then pushing up on the prolapsed bladder. This can help any residual urine move up closer to the uretheral opening. Yes, it's a bit more messy, but also very effective.

Avoid Bladder Infections After Sex

Worried about bladder infections following sexual activity? We know that the force of urine flow helps wash away bacteria that may be trying to migrate up to the bladder and can cause an infection. However, you don't have to jump up right after sex and rush to the bathroom, which can impact the sexy mood and really dampen romance. It's okay to wait a half hour or so, and then leisurely make your way to use the bathroom to urinate and wipe away extra lubrication and secretions.

REGAINING DRYNESS

Fortunately, there's a range of treatment options that can help you become dry or drier. Who wants to visit every bathroom every thirty minutes or spend a fortune on pads? Now you don't have to. Many women haven't heard about the most effective treatments and are surprised when they're suggested. Many women do not need surgery and can be helped with pelvic-floor physical therapy.

My goal for any woman who is leaking is to improve the situation, decrease the number of visits to the bathroom, and work toward complete dryness. However, if leaking is extensive, even a 50 to 75 percent improvement can make a powerful and positive difference in how we enjoy our lives. Don't be afraid to bring this up during a visit to your healthcare practitioner. Talk about any leaking you might have and ask about pelvic-floor physical therapy classes, a certified pelvic-floor physical therapist, and medications that might help. If you're considering surgery, be sure to get a second opinion from a urologist or urogynecologist.

14

Standing Tall and Straight with Healthy Bones

$\mathcal{T}$he idea of a hot and sexy menopause conjures up a vision of a self-assured woman striding confidently through life. She's able to stand up straight, walk without a limp, and isn't hunched over. The truth is how we care for our bones during menopause will affect our lives for decades to come. In menopause, though, we have lots of other more immediate concerns, keeping our bones strong and healthy is one of the most important preventive measures we can take right now. Avoiding significant height loss and preventing fractures help women continue to live their lives without restrictions and pain.

Although our bones would seem to be like rocks or steel, never changing, the truth is that our bones are in a dynamic and constant state of change. Like interior decorators, who are always improving upon the appearance of a room, our bones, too, are perpetually remodeling. As older bone is replaced with newer bone, our bodies continue the constant process of bone renewal. Estrogen is one of the key factors in helping our bodies build strong, new bone to replace old bone that is lost. Diets rich in calcium, vitamin D, magnesium, and other nutrients are also important in helping our bones attain their maximal density in our late teens and early twenties. Between the twenties and forties, when estrogen levels are relatively stable, most women's bone density and strength are relatively stable. The one exception is found at another time when estrogen levels decline—during breast-feeding. That bone loss, however, is rapidly replaced when a woman stops nursing.

In menopause, hormonal changes lead to decreased bone mass. As estrogen levels decline, more bone is lost than our bodies are able to rebuild. Women can lose up to 20 percent of their bone mass in the first five to seven years after menopause. Estrogen is one of the most important hormones that help our bones stay strong. When estrogen levels decrease, bone mass also decreases. As more bone is lost, the bones aren't as able to support weight and are more likely to fracture. The first sign of bone loss is often a loss in height of one or more inches. No one wants to lose height, or worse, fracture a bone, so keeping our bones healthy in menopause and beyond helps increase the likelihood that we'll be able to enjoy all our normal activities without pain or the worry of falling and breaking a bone.

Having a cool and sexy menopause also means being able to walk confidently into a room, and that means having strong and healthy bones. There are so many questions and so much confusion around bone health in menopause that I'd like to introduce three women—Elise, Dana, and Patti—who represent a range of bone-health scenarios.

ELISE'S STORY

Elise's wedding was lovely. She had waited a long time to meet a guy like Ted, who was thoughtful, smart, and loved to travel. In a few days, they would be flying off to Hawaii for a honeymoon. Her friends were all giving Elise ideas about beaches and restaurants, while I was urging her to take a helicopter tour of the remote Na Pali coast on the island of Kauai. "I'd be too nervous to fly around it, so we're hiking that trail," she laughed. "I just want to lie on the beach and drink mai tais."

My husband and I headed back to California after the wedding, thinking of Elise and Ted on their honeymoon with palm trees, warm surf, and yes, mai tais. I wasn't prepared for the shocking call I received at 3 AM about a week later. It was Elise calling from Hawaii, and it took me a minute to register what she was saying between sobs.

Elise and Ted had been hiking on the famous Na Pali coast just that day, when Elise fell down. She knew that there was something very wrong. Ted flagged down some other hikers to get help. After what seemed like for-

ever, park rangers came up the trail and called for a helicopter. Elise did get a helicopter tour, but she was on a gurney with a paramedic at her side. "I didn't see much," she said. "I was so scared, I couldn't open my eyes."

Elise was transported to a hospital where x-rays confirmed the diagnosis of a fractured hip. She was only forty-seven. Elise had four pins placed during her hip surgery and recovered in a hospital for the last few days of her honeymoon in Hawaii. When she returned home, her doctor ordered a battery of tests including a bone mineral density test—called a dual-energy x-ray absorptiometry (DEXA) scan—which revealed that she had severe osteoporosis and severe bone loss. As Elise recuperated, she wrote thank-you notes, practiced walking on crutches, and spent four months in intense physical therapy and rehabilitation. She was able to work from home for a while and eventually made a full recovery.

Elise's story is dramatic, but there's a lot we can all learn from her experience. She had a strong family history of osteoporosis, many of her older aunts were stooped and hunched over, and her seventy-two-year-old mother was taking osteoporosis medication.

Elise never drank milk and only occasionally had cheese. Her vitamin D level was 19 ng/ml, well below the recommended 32 ng/ml. Elise was not close to perimenopause or menopause. Her periods came regularly. Her osteoporosis and fractured hip were not a result of menopause; she had very low bone density to begin with. However, she would be at an even greater risk as she went through menopause for more bone loss and fractures.

Here are Elise's bone mineral density results from the DEXA scan, which are reported as negative T scores:

Lumbar Spine T: –3.3 (osteoporosis)

Hip T: –3.7 (osteoporosis)

Here is the range of DEXA T-score results that testing reveals, along with their meanings:

T = 0 to –1.0 (Normal; low risk of fracture)

T = –1.0 to –2.5 (Osteopenia; mild bone loss)

T = –2.5 and lower (Osteoporosis; increased risk of hip and spine fractures)

Elise's T scores were negative 3.3 and 3.7, which are lower than negative 2.5 and indicate that she has osteoporosis.

Elise's doctor recommended an oral bisphosphonate medication, Actonel, which helped her improve her bone density and reduced the risk of having another fracture. She was also advised to start increasing her calcium intake and was prescribed 2,000 IU of vitamin D each day. Within two years, Elise's bone mineral density values had improved, and I'm happy to say that, after six years, she has not lost any height and hasn't fractured any other bones.

DANA'S STORY

Dana's story was not quite so dramatic. A fifty-seven-year old woman who came to see me as a new patient, Dana needed her annual exam and wanted to talk about options for treating her worsening vaginal dryness. She hadn't had a period in four years and was never bothered by hot flashes or night sweats. Dana was a woman who seemed to have found balance in her life. She was happily married and was able to spend her time gardening, walking the dog, and volunteering at a local hospital. She also played in a tennis league and occasionally got in a round of golf on weekends.

Dana was very interested in staying healthy. She didn't smoke, rarely drank, and tried to follow the advice of her healthcare providers as long as it made sense.

She was on thyroid medication for her hypothyroidism and rarely needed something for the migraines that occurred one to two times a year. Dana took calcium and vitamin D supplements every day because her lactose intolerance meant that drinking milk led to bloating, cramps, and gas.

The first way I test for bone loss is to measure height. Dana was 5 feet, 7 inches, exactly what she had been since high school. We then talked about menopause issues from A to Z. Her thyroid disease was a risk factor for bone loss, and a bone density test three years previously showed osteopenia, which is mild bone loss and meant that she needed close monitoring. I asked her to have another bone density test in addition to checking cholesterol and vitamin D levels and having thyroid tests.

Dana's vitamin D level was 48, which meant that all the time out of doors was helping her absorb enough sunlight to convert plenty of vitamin

D. Her bone mineral density was about the same as it was three years ago, which was reassuring.

Here are Dana's bone density results, reported as negative T scores:

Dana's first bone density test results:

Lumbar Spine T: *−1.2 (osteopenia)*

Hip T: *−0.8 (normal)*

Dana's second bone density test results:

Lumbar Spine T: *−1.3 (osteopenia)*

Hip T: *−0.9 (normal)*

Dana's T scores were virtually the same at the second testing, with only a slight difference in the lumbar spine. Her results were in the normal range for her hip and only showed mild bone loss, osteopenia, in her lumbar spine. What was more reassuring was that Dana was four years from her last period and still had almost the same bone density. She was in great shape. Her weight-bearing exercise and adequate calcium and vitamin D intake were all contributing to her healthy bones and counteracting any negative effects of the thyroid disease. I advised her to continue all of her healthy habits and we'd recheck in two to three years.

PATTI'S STORY

Patti was a new patient who came to see me shortly after moving back to her hometown to care for her elderly parents. As a consultant, she could work anywhere near a major airport and moved back to her family home. Patti sailed through menopause three years earlier without many symptoms. She was a bit breathless as she described arranging for in-home caregivers for her dad, who had Alzheimer's disease, and her mom, who had just been released from a rehab facility after breaking a hip.

Patti's stress level was off the charts. She coped with her new role as a caregiver with red wine and dark chocolate. "I'm a little worried," she confided. "I think I'm drinking too much. It's definitely a crutch right now." After getting her folks settled for the night and briefing the night nurse, she would retreat to her room to watch old movies with a bag of chocolate candy and a bottle of red wine to help her sleep.

The added stress also sparked a nasty case of shingles, which was treated with an antiviral and steroids for ten days. Though this short expo-sure to steroids was a slight concern for her bone health, it wasn't as risky as taking steroids for three months would have been. The bigger risk fac-tors for her bones were her family history and her alcohol intake.

Patti's lab tests showed that her liver was functioning normally, but her vitamin D level was low at 20 (ng/ml), lower than what we'd like to see (32 ng/ml), and her bone mineral density revealed significant bone loss. Like her mother, Patti had osteoporosis, meaning that she, too, had a greater risk of a fracture.

Here are Patti's bone mineral density test results, reported as negative T scores:

Lumbar Spine T: −3.1 (osteoporosis)

Hip T: −2.8 (osteoporosis)

Patti's T scores were both lower than negative 2.5 and thus she had osteoporosis of both her lumbar spine and her hip.

I plugged Patti's bone mineral density results into the FRAX calculator that's recommended by the World Health Organization. This uses a woman's bone mineral density readings, her age, race, family history, and other risk factors to predict the risk of fracture in ten years. Patti's risk factors were her alcohol use and her family history. According to the FRAX charts, her risk of fracture in ten years was approximately 25 percent. That meant that she had a 1 in 4 chance that she would suffer a fracture within ten years. After caring for her mom, she was ready to discuss her treatment options.

I strongly recommended that she decrease her alcohol intake and in-crease calcium intake and weight-bearing exercise. I also prescribed 50,000 international units (IU) of vitamin D to take each week, and suggested that she start medication to help her body rebuild bone. She started on an oral tablet, Boniva, which she took once each month.

Patti's most recent bone mineral density test showed a marked improve-ment in both her spine and hip, reducing her risk of fracturing in the future.

THE NITTY-GRITTY ON OUR BONES

Collectively, our bones make up our frame or skeleton, which supports our weight. Bone that appears rock solid is actually a network of interlacing supports. And though bone is hard and strong, it's constantly in a state of remodeling or turnover. Old bone is removed by osteoclasts, while new bone is added by osteoblasts. Our bones stay healthy and strong by keeping a balance between what's being broken down and removed and what's being built back up. Bone health is also influenced by the amount of calcium, vitamin D, magnesium, and other nutrients that are available for rebuilding healthy bone.

Before a woman enters perimenopause, the estrogen produced by her ovaries enables her bones to stay strong and healthy. Yet as estrogen levels decline, bone mass also declines. In and around menopause, the amount of bone loss from osteoclastic activity exceeds the amount of bone buildup by the osteoblasts, producing a net loss of bone. In fact, women can lose up to 20 percent of their bone mass in the first five to seven years after menopause.

Why Weight-Bearing Exercise Is Important

For our bones to be strong, we have to use them. Standing upright, supporting our weight, and walking is best for our bones and every other system in our bodies. We're healthiest when we're moving. Study after study on people confined to their beds has shown that bone density melts away when people aren't upright and moving. Likewise, NASA found the same result with astronauts in zero gravity. When floating around without bearing any weight, bone density decreases.

Studies also show that walking, running, dancing, cycling, gardening, and all other forms of weight-bearing exercise strengthen our bones. Just standing up sends signals the bone to be stronger. Clearly our bones are happiest when we're up moving around, bearing our own weight. Despite all their best efforts, there are many women who lose bone mass after menopause from the loss of estrogen. They do everything right, exercise, get plenty of calcium, have adequate vitamin D, don't drink or smoke, and still they may be losing enough bone to be at risk for a fracture. Luckily, there are effective treatments available and prevention strategies that can help our bones be their healthiest.

. . . .

Risk Factors for Bone Loss

- Family history of osteoporosis
- Personal history of fracture as an adult
- Menopause
- Recent falls
- A lifetime history of low-calcium intake
- Little physical exercise
- Smoking
- High caffeine intake—more than three servings/day
- Excessive alcohol—three or more drinks/day
- Loss of periods from surgical menopause
- Anorexia or low body weight
- Use of some medications—steroids, anticonvulsants, insulin, thyroid medication
- Low vitamin D levels

. . . .

TESTING, TESTING, TESTING

The following are guidelines from the National Osteoporosis Foundation (NOF) on who should have bone mineral density (BMD) testing. BMD tests are recommended for:

- Women sixty-five and older
- Men seventy and older
- People who have broken a bone after age fifty
- Women who are menopausal with any risk factors
- Women between menopause and age sixty-five with risk factors

Consider BMD testing when there has been:

- An x-ray that shows bone loss or a break in the bones of the spine

- Back pain with possible break in any bones of the spine

- A loss of one-half inch or more of height within one year

- A loss of one and one-half inches of height from a person's maximal height

Bone Mineral Density Testing

It's been my experience that virtually every woman has at least one risk factor for bone loss around menopause. If possible, and if insurance covers the test, I recommend a baseline bone mineral density test at menopause and then another one every two to three years depending upon each woman's situation. I like having a snapshot of where a woman's bone mass is at menopause, since that level is likely to be as good as it's ever going to be. Most women will see their bone mass decline by as much as 20 percent within the first five to seven years after menopause.

- **PERIPHERAL TESTS.** Peripheral tests use ultrasound to measure the bone density at the heel or wrist. Not as accurate as the DEXA outlined below. Because the machine is small and can be done just about anywhere, this is often a good first start to identify people who may need further testing.

- **DEXA OR DXA (DUAL ENERGY X-RAY ABSORPTIOMETRY).** This is a simple, painless, fifteen-minute test that measures the bone density of the hip and spine. The bone density is compared to that of a healthy thirty-five-year-old women. DEXA results are given in negative (–) T scores. The following are DEXA T scores and their meanings:

T = 0 to -1.0	Normal; low risk of fracture
T = -1.0 to -2.5	Osteopenia; mild bone loss
T = -2.5 and lower	Osteoporosis; increased risk of hip and spine fractures

Blood Tests for Vitamin D levels

Known as the sunshine vitamin because our skin utilizes ultraviolet light to make it, vitamin D is an essential nutrient for bone health. Blood levels should be at least 32 ng/ml or higher. Studies on surfers in Hawaii who weren't using sunscreen found a range of vitamin D levels, but most maxed out at 70 ng/ml. Many experts are advising people to aim for levels around 40 ng/ml.

People at risk for vitamin D deficiency:

- Have very little sun exposure

- Use sunscreen or cover up when outside

- Have celiac disease, Crohn's disease, or other conditions that interfere with the absorption of nutrients

- Have had gastric bypass surgery, which interferes with the absorption of nutrients

- Take medications that can interfere with vitamin D absorption, such as epilepsy medications

- Have darker skins and need more time in sunlight to make vitamin D

- Live in colder northern latitudes, which makes it more difficult to get prolonged sun exposure in winter

SIMPLE STEPS TO HEALTHIER BONES

The best way to prevent bone loss is to get plenty of calcium, vitamin D, and other nutrients for bone health. This means a varied diet with plenty of vegetables, fish, protein, and dairy.

Calcium-Rich Food

Recent evidence has confirmed what many studies have shown in the past. I'm all about food first, and it's preferable for women to get their calcium from a balanced diet. Dairy products such as milk, yogurt, cheese, cottage cheese, and even ice cream are all good sources of calcium. There's also calcium in sardines, almonds, and green leafy vegetables such as spinach, collard greens, kale, and broccoli.

What About Lactose Intolerance?

Between one-third and one-half of women around the age of menopause believe they have a lactose intolerance, meaning they lack the enzyme, lactase, that helps break down the milk sugar known as lactose. This leads to gas, bloating, and in some cases, diarrhea. Many people who believe that they are lactose intolerant are actually lactose sensitive, which means that they are able to tolerate limited amounts of dairy without stomach upset. Ounce for ounce, milk has more lactose than yogurt or cheese, so people who are lactose sensitive may find that they can enjoy those foods with few to no symptoms.

Some women have successfully increased their dairy consumption and overcome what they though was a lactose intolerance by gradually increasing the amount of dairy they take in. I start my patients on yogurt, since the beneficial bacteria, lactobacilli and bifidobacteria, seem to help create a more acid environment in the tummy, helping to minimize the lactose intolerance. In addition to yogurt and cheese, which both have less lactose than milk, I recommend Lactaid milk and Lactaid tablets as another good option to get plenty of calcium. See the end of the chapter for a step-by-step program to help increase your dairy if you're lactose sensitive.

Calcium Supplements

I routinely recommend calcium supplements to women who aren't able to get three servings of calcium-rich foods each day. Women who do have adequate calcium in their diet do not need added supplements. Research on a possible association between calcium supplements and heart disease has led to the recommendation that women should consume up to 800 milligrams (mg) of calcium in supplements each day but not more than that.

Vitamin D Sources

Vitamin D is essential, not only for optimal calcium absorption, but also has been associated with reduced risks of breast and colon cancer. Most Caucasians need about ten to fifteen minutes of sunlight each day before they lather on the sunscreen. Darker-skinned people need more time in the sun. For people who live in northern latitudes, it's important to get lots of sun in the summer time, since vitamin D is a fat-soluble vitamin and will be stored in their fat until colder, darker months. Other sources of vitamin D include fatty fish such as wild salmon, mackerel, tuna, sardines, and cod, as well as vitamin D–fortified cow's milk and soy milk. Maybe it's not just the bitter cold weather in the north that sends people heading south for the winter; it could be that their bodies are craving more vitamin D.

Vitamin D Supplements

Consider taking a vitamin D supplement in the darker winter months if you suspect that you're deficient from lack of sun exposure or if you have celiac disease. For patients with a severe vitamin D deficiency, I often prescribe 50,000 IU once each week to get their levels up to 32 ng/ml. For women with a slight deficiency, often 1,000 to 2,000 IU/day will suffice.

Magnesium

Magnesium is also important for maintaining bone health. Although most people get adequate magnesium in their diet if they eat at least two to three servings of fruits and vegetables each day, there are people at risk for lower magnesium levels. People with type 2 diabetes, with gastrointestinal issues, people who've had gastric surgery, or those who drink more than two alcoholic drinks per day are at risk for low magnesium levels. According to the National Institutes of Health, the recommended amount of magnesium for women over thirty is 320 mg daily.

Other Important Nutrients for Bone Health

A diet with a variety of fruits and vegetables that include every color and type imaginable, from potatoes, tomatoes, strawberries, papaya, and broccoli to Brussels sprouts, red, green, and yellow peppers, and all the greens you can eat will provide vitamin K, vitamin C, potassium, and the other essential nutrients for bone health. The key to getting all the essential nutrients is to aim for variety and multiple colors on the plate.

Supplements and Multivitamins

Despite their best efforts, many people just can't manage to get the recommended five to seven servings of fruits and vegetables each day, plus three servings of dairy. It may also be a bit daunting to eat two servings of fatty fish each week. I'm all about food first, but I'm also a realist. Many people, including myself, take supplements to round out the gaps in our diet. What's important to remember is not to take more than is recommended and to continue to eat a variety of nutritious food.

I recommend multivitamins daily or a few times each week to anyone who doesn't have a balanced diet and isn't getting at least three servings of fruits and vegetables each day. I don't count fruit juice as a serving, but vegetable or tomato juice does count. I advise people to look for a multivitamin that has no more than 100 percent of the daily recommended amounts of nutrients; otherwise, they're paying for vitamins that aren't getting absorbed.

Exercise

Everyone needs to exercise regularly. It's essential for every aspect of maintaining a healthy body and a healthy mind. I hope that you're already exercising regularly, and if so, please take a look at whether you're getting enough work with weights, stretching, and resistance training. If you're not exercising as much as you know you should, don't give up and get overwhelmed by the idea. You're not alone. There are an infinite number of barriers and excuses that prevent people from exercising, I know because I've not only heard them all but I've also used them myself. It's important to start with honesty and an awareness of what's preventing you from moving regularly.

Then make a plan that you can commit to. Maybe it's as simple as walking around the block once each day for five minutes. You might also use a pedometer to see how many steps you take each day, then aim for 5,000 steps, which is the minimum amount each of us should be getting. Gradually, you can work up to 10,000 steps each day, which is a great way to improve your overall health. Many of my patients erroneously assume that they have to work out strenuously or there's no benefit. The truth is this: Any and all movement is beneficial. Walking for ten minutes a day is a good start.

My advice for people who haven't exercised in a while is to start slowly and set a personal goal. If there's no time for a thirty-minute walk, don't throw in the towel. Instead, be happy you got ten minutes. Any minutes of exercise is better than none. Sometimes we think in terms of "all or nothing." As people get up and get moving it gets easier to get motivated the next time. We realize that a brisk walk is not so bad after all and that we feel lots better afterward. This also applies to those of us who have an exercise routine. I know there are days when I have to motivate myself to get off the couch and walk the dog. The point is to get up, find something you enjoy, and then do it regularly. If you have joint pain or are immobile, talk to your healthcare practitioner about physical therapy so that you can regain your mobility. And if you don't find anything you like, you're not trying hard enough.

Ask yourself these questions to help make a realistic exercise plan:

- How much time do you have to exercise?

- How long can you walk now?

- Where will you go?

- Do you have a friend to exercise with?

- Does the weather affect your exercise routine?

- Is your neighborhood safe to walk in?

Medications for Healthier Bones

Women at menopause often don't need medication for bone loss. Their risk of fracture is lower than for women who are ten or more years older, when the risk of fracture increases. For women at menopause with risk factors, there are a variety of prescription medications available to treat their bone loss. Younger women can often be treated for three to five years and then take a "holiday" from the medications since these meds have long-lasting beneficial effects.

Bisphosphonates

There are oral and intravenous (IV) bisphosphonate formulations.

Oral preparations include Actonel (risedronate), Boniva (ibandronate), Fosamax (alendronate), and Reclast (zoledronic acid). These nonhormonal prescription medications all reduce the risk of hip and spinal fracture by approximately 50 percent in three years. They work to reduce bone loss by inhibiting the osteoclasts from breaking down as much bone, which allows the osteoblasts to catch up and build more bone.

Among these products, there are weekly and monthly formulations. These medications are difficult to absorb, so they must be taken on an empty stomach and the person must remain upright for at least thirty minutes.

Possible side effects with all of the oral medications include stomach upset and irritation of the esophagus.

For these medications to work properly, it is also essential to have plenty of the building blocks we need for bone formation, including a diet that's rich in calcium and protein and having adequate exposure to vitamin D.

IV bisphosphonates include Boniva (ibandronate) and Reclast (zole-dronic acid). Boniva is given by IV every three months. Reclast is given once a year. These reduce the risk of fracture between 50 to 70 percent in three years. Side effects include flulike symptoms for a few days. For people with certain bone cancers who use IV bisphosphonates, there have been rare instances of osteonecrosis of the jaw, where the bone that supports the teeth starts to degrade, leading to loss of bone and teeth.

Parathyroid Hormone

Forteo (teriparatide) is an expensive daily injection that stimulates new bone formation. It was found to increase bone mass by 9.7 percent in the spine and by 2.6 percent in the hip. This is an option for someone with severe bone loss, with T scores less than -4.0, or who might not tolerate the other medications. Side effects include pain, muscle aches, dizziness, and runny noses.

Rank Ligand Inhibitor

Prolia (denosumab) is a new class of medication to treat osteoporosis. It is given as a subcutaneous injection every six months. Prolia completely suppresses the osteoclasts that break down bone. In three years the fracture reduction is 40 percent in the hip and 68 percent in the spine. Side effects include back pain, muscle pain, infections of the skin and urinary tract, and eczema. There have been rare reports of osteonecrosis of the jaw, where the bone that supports the teeth starts to degrade, leading to loss of bone and teeth.

· ·

Nurse Barb's Tummy-Soothing Lactose Sensitivity Tips

When trying to increase dairy, if you believe you have an underlying lactose intolerance, don't have dairy by itself. Always try to have some other food along with your small trial of yogurt, cheese, or milk. The addition of other food will help the intestine adjust to any lactose that's present. Lactaid milk is another option, as there's no lactose in it.

Here's a program that I developed for my patients to increase their dairy.

• For the first two weeks, have one level teaspoon of yogurt with active cultures with each meal every day.

• In weeks two through four, increase yogurt to two teaspoons at each meal.

• If there are any intestinal symptoms, go back to one teaspoon at each meal.

- In weeks four through six, try one level tablespoon of yogurt each day ($^1/_2$ ounce).

- In weeks six through eight, try two level tablespoons of yogurt each day (1 ounce).

- After week eight, try $^1/_2$ cup of yogurt a few times each week.

- If $^1/_2$ cup of yogurt is tolerated, then most people can tolerate a few sips of Lactaid or one small piece of cheese.

- If possible, slowly work up to 1 cup of yogurt a few times per week and $^1/_2$ cup of Lactaid or cheese at meals.

- If there are any intestinal symptoms go back to the level of dairy that was tolerated.

- If you're unable to have two to three servings of dairy, then do start taking a calcium supplement with vitamin D.

Nurse Barb's Hot Exercise Tips

- Find a friend to exercise with or walk your dog—time flies with a buddy.

- Distraction can help you forget your resistance; work out with an iPod, music, or TV.

- Try water aerobics; though there's no weight bearing, the resistance from the water is a good start.

- Swimming or using a kickboard for a few laps may be a good option for women with back pain.

- Yoga is a great option, not just for the improved flexibility that helps keep joints pliable and moving in all directions, but for the yoga breathing that has been shown to decrease the severity and number of hot flashes.

- Pilates is another superb option for strength and flexibility and helps work muscles that have been in hiding and underused.

- Dance classes improve balance and coordination, making falls less likely.

- If you start exercising five minutes each day, the goal is to work up to thirty minutes each day at least six times every week. This will not only strengthen your bones but also decrease the risk of heart disease, obesity, diabetes, breast cancer, and colon cancer.

- Weight training is also an important aspect of any exercise routine. Thirty minutes, three times a week is an ideal start.

- One of the big secrets of weight training is that it builds more muscle, which helps to burn more fat.

- Use one-pound ankle weights to get weight training simultaneously with your daily activities. It will help jump-start weight loss and really tones the legs.

STAND TALL

Bone health is a hidden but important aspect of health at every age, but during menopause it becomes especially important to work on healthy habits to prevent fractures later in life. Having a hot and sexy menopause means standing up straight and tall and doing everything you can to stay that way so that you can enjoy your life to it's fullest. The easiest way to have healthy bones is to get regular exercise, plenty of calcium and vitamin D, and maintain a healthy diet rich in nutrients.

Conclusion

*M*enopause and midlife are two of the most important transitions that a woman will make. This is a time of profound personal growth combined with what may seem like overwhelming physical and emotional changes. Every woman's experience is unique, yet there are some commonalities that we all share. I know that each woman must find her own path, which is why I've offered real stories from real women, plus a peek into the solutions they found most helpful with their own menopausal challenges. My patients are always telling me what's most important to them, and I have tried to share their experiences and questions with you. My goal was to infuse the stories with humor, so that we sidestep getting overwhelmed, laugh about some of the most vexing issues we deal with, and then solve them in ways you may not have considered.

We need to know what's coming up for us, not with dread but with knowledge and empowerment. We need to know that, if we want it, a hot and sexy menopause is within our reach. We need to know that, yes, we're normal, and yes, everything is going to be just fine. Wait, not just fine, but so much better than we ever expected. We need to know that we can design our own unique journey, the one that fits us best, which is why I included all sorts of secret tips and sexy tips and tips that cover everything from your skin and hair to how to have better sex and even how to lose some weight.

This truly is the time to celebrate all the wonderful accumulated wisdom you have gathered through the years, to tap into your strengths, and to stride confidently along this journey. I hope you'll find here all the knowledge, and above all, the empowerment, to find what works best for you so that you can have a cool, sexy menopause! Really.

APPENDIX

Some Insight into the Studies on Hormones

Women's Health Initiative (WIH) Study

With all the controversies swirling around hormone treatments for peri-menopausal and menopausal women, it may be beneficial to go back and look at some of our old assumptions about hormones, and then look at what newer research has found since the Women's Health Initiative (WIH) study results were first reported in 2002.

The WHI study was designed to look at whether estrogen and progesterone, in the form of the most commonly prescribed formulations Premarin and PremPro, not only reduced hot flashes and night sweats but also had a protective effect for heart disease. It was a valid question to ask, because heart disease is responsible for about half of all deaths in women after menopause. Previous research had shown that estrogen had some protective effects on preventing atherosclerotic plaque buildup in carotid arteries and maintaining cardiovascular health. Was estrogen keeping the heart and the arteries healthy? It seemed plausible that the same estrogen hormones that reduced hot flashes and night sweats, improving quality of life, might also prevent heart disease. Researchers were also interested in estrogen's association with breast cancer.

Prior to 2002, there was a lot of conflicting research on the effects of estrogen on breast cancer and cardiovascular disease, which made the WHI results, with over 160,000 women studied, even more powerful. When the results showed an unexpected increased risk of breast cancer, stroke, blood clots, and cardiovascular disease, it was a bitter and deeply disappointing pill to swallow. Though the Nurses' Health Study and Nurses' Health Study II (ongoing since 1976) showed similar breast cancer rates, many researchers, clinicians, and women were shocked.

No matter what other research has shown, the FDA ruled that all estrogens and progesterone options for menopausal remedies must carry the same warnings based on the findings from the WHI.

The results of the WHI didn't make sense to many clinicians because in their experience, the vast majority of women who used hormones had no serious side effects. However, if we put on our CSI detective hats and look at this issue from a different vantage point, it starts to make more sense. The fact is, most providers and nurse practitioners, even those in large group practices, only have 1,000 to 5,000 patients in their practice—a fraction of the number studied in the WHI. In their day-to-day practice, they rarely had a patient on hormones who had experienced a serious adverse event. It didn't make sense to them until much larger numbers of women were compiled. With 50,000 and 100,000 to 160,000 women studied, suddenly the evidence revealed itself.

The WHI reported results in 10,000 woman-years. This simply means that they analyzed what happened when hormones were taken for one year's time in 10,000 women. This takes into account women on hormones for six months and those on it for more than one year.

The WHI found that for every 10,000 woman-years, for those who took a combination of estrogen and progesterone in the form of Prem-Pro, there were:

- 7 more cardiovascular events, such as heart attacks

- 8 more strokes

- 8 more clots in the lungs (pulmonary embolism)

- 8 more breast cancers

- 6 fewer colorectal cancers

- 5 fewer hip fractures

Clearly, the assumption that estrogen would prevent heart disease was erroneous. Instead of preventing heart disease, women over sixty years of age, those with high blood pressure, and those who smoked not only *didn't* benefit from starting estrogen, they had a higher probability of being harmed by taking it.

But the Women's Health Initiative (WHI) study, reported in 2002, had many problematic issues, including:

- Only Premarin and Prempro were studied, the most popular types of hormone treatments available at the time the study began.

- Premarin is an oral form of estrogen and is conjugated equine estrogen.

- Premarin is derived from a "natural" source, that is, the urine of pregnant horses (mares). Hence the name: **PRE**gnant **MAR**e's ur**IN**e.

- PremPro contains Premarin and Provera, a synthetic progestin (medroxyprogesterone acetate), with some of the properties of progesterone and the ability to be absorbed orally.

- Though the study included women in their early fifties, most of the women studied were much older, in their mid- to late sixties.

- The study also included women who started hormones more than five years after menopause, which we learned from this study increases the risks named in the study.

- 10 percent of women in the study smoked.

- Approximately 25 percent of the women in the study had high blood pressure.

- The study was stopped after there were too many breast cancers observed in the group on Prempro.

But what about younger women in their early fifties? Did age make a difference in risk for the cardiovascular events such as blood clots, stroke, and heart attacks? What about women who had normal cholesterol levels and who hadn't already developed atherosclerotic plaques in their coronary arteries? Would they benefit from estrogen as the data from other studies suggested?

In addition, was the type of estrogen and progesterone the culprit? What if other types of hormones were used? Was it possible that the way the hormones were absorbed made a difference in risk, either orally from a pill or through the skin from a patch, cream, or gel? What if there were different types of estrogen and progesterone molecules? Would the results be the same?

From the perspective of the average clinician, it seemed that breast cancer was just as prevalent in women on both estrogen and progesterone as women not taking them. And yet the evidence from both the Nurses' Health Study and the WHI lined up. Taking hormones after menopause does seem to accelerate the growth of undetectable breast cancers and increases the risk of breast cancer. For every 100 women who do not take hormones, approximately 2 will be diagnosed with breast cancer in a year. For women who do take hormones, 3 will be diagnosed with breast cancer in a year.

The Women's Health Initiative (WHI) Revisited

Since the results of the WHI study were first reported, there has been follow-up research reported on the younger women in the study who were healthier, had no cardiovascular risk factors, and started hormones earlier. The consensus is that these women have *less* risk of cardiovascular disease than women who forgo hormone treatment. This has led to the "estrogen timing hypothesis," which means that early use may be beneficial in helping to delay and prevent cardiovascular risk. This may be very important for women who undergo a surgical menopause from having their ovaries removed and for women who start menopause in their forties.

The caveat is that estrogen and progesterone therapies should not be used as a prevention or as a treatment for cardiovascular disease because of the harm that could result. Also, women who are five or more years past menopause should not start hormone treatment. In all cases, it's important to discuss your personal medical and family history with your own licensed healthcare provider to get the best individualized advice for your unique situation.

The KEEPS Trial

In July 2012, results from a four-year study on over 700 women were announced. The Kronos Early Estrogen Progesterone Study (KEEPS) looked at a number of the risks identified with hormone use by the WHI. The researchers studied differences in women using no hormones, those on a low dose of Premarin, and a low dose of the Climara estrogen patch. Additionally, unlike the WHI, where women took Provera, in the KEEPs trial, women who had a uterus also received a bioidentical progesterone, Prometrium. Though over 700 women were studied, far fewer than in the WHI, these were younger women, they didn't smoke, didn't have high blood pressure, and they were followed for four years. The results are encouraging for women and healthcare providers about the use of estrogen within the first three years of menopause.

When considering the risk of cardiovascular disease, there were no differences in the rate of coronary artery atherosclerosis progression in any of the women regardless of whether they used hormones or which ones they used. This was determined using coronary artery calcium scores (CACs). There was also no increased rates of blood clots, stroke, or breast cancer in the study. The authors cautioned that, while these results were encouraging, the small size of the study meant that we couldn't draw definitive conclusions. However, for younger, healthy women with hot flashes and night sweats, the KEEPS trial may help them worry less about serious risks.

Though there's no consensus on whether using hormones for hot flashes and night sweats improves sex drive, libido, and sexual response, many women find that they're more interested in sex after starting hormone treatment. Whether it's the improved sleep or the hormonal influences on arousal, many women have been pleasantly surprised by the return of their sex drive. The KEEPS trial also found that women on both low-dose oral estrogen and transdermal estrogen enjoyed more lubrication and less pain. There were also significant improvements in desire and arousal for the women on transdermal estrogen.

References

Allison, M. A., et al. "Oophorectomy, hormone therapy, and subclinical coronary artery disease in women with hysterectomy: The Women's Health Initiative coronary artery calcium study." *Menopause,* 2008 Jul–Aug; 15 (4 Pt, 1): 639–47.

Aso, T., et al. "A natural S-equol supplement alleviates hot flushes and other menopausal symptoms in equol nonproducing postmenopausal Japanese women." *J Womens Health,* 2012 Jan; 21 (1): 92–100.

Borud, E. K., et al. "The acupuncture on hot flushes among menopausal women (ACUFLASH) study: A randomized controlled trial." *Menopause,* 2009 May–Jun; 16 (3): 484–93.

Eden J. A., N. F. Hacker, and M. Fortune. "Three cases of endometrial cancer associated with 'bioidentical' hormone replacement therapy." *Med J Aust,* 2007; 187 (4): 244–45.

Harman, S. M., et al. "Is the WHI relevant to HRT started in perimenopause?" *Endocrine,* 2004 Aug; 24 (3): 195–202.

Jenks, B. H., et al. "A pilot study on the effects of S-equol compared to soy isoflavones on menopausal hot flash frequency." *J Womens Health,* 2012 Jun; 21 (6): 674–82.

Kang, W., et al. "Effect of soy isoflavones on breast cancer recurrence and death on patients receiving adjuvant endocrine therapy." *CMAJ,* 2010; 182: 1857–62.

Klok, M. D., et al. "The role of leptin and ghrelin in the regulation of food intake and body weight in humans: A review." *Obes Rev,* 2007 Jan; 8 (1): 21–34.

Labrie, F., et al. "Intravaginal dehydroepiandrosterone (Prasterone), a physiological and highly efficient treatment of vaginal atrophy." *Menopause,* 2009 Sep–Oct; 16 (5): 907–22.

Manson, J. E., et al. "Estrogen therapy and coronary-artery calcification." *N Engl J Med,* 2007 Jun 21; 356 (25): 2591–602.

Manson, J. E., et al. "Postmenopausal hormone therapy: New questions and the case for new clinical trials." *Menopause,* 2006 Jan–Feb; 13 (1): 139–47.

Messina, M., D. I. Abrams, and M. Hardy. "Can clinicians now assure their breast cancer patients that soy foods are safe?" *Womens Health (Lon Engl),* 2010; 6: 335–8.

Naftolin, F., et al. "The Women's Health Initiative could not have detected cardioprotective effects of starting hormone therapy during the menopause transition." *Fertil Steril,* 2004 Jun; 81 (6): 1498–501.

North American Menopause Society, Hormone Position Statement, 2012. Retrieved from www.NAMS.org.

Pinkerton, J. V., et al. "Bazedoxifene/conjugated estrogens for menopausal symptom treatment and osteoporosis prevention." *Climacteric,* 2012 Oct; 15 (5): 411–8.

Portman, D. J., et al. "Ospemifene, a novel selective estrogen receptor modulator for treating dyspareunia associated with postmenopausal vulvar and vaginal atrophy." *Menopause,* 2013 Jun; 20 (6): 623–30.

Rossouw, J. E., et al. "Postmenopausal hormone therapy and risk of cardiovascular disease by age and years since menopause." *JAMA,* 2007 Apr 4; 297 (13): 1465–77.

Rossouw, J. E., et al.: Writing group for the Women's Health Initiative Investigators. "Risks and benefits of estrogen plus progestin in healthy postmenopausal women: Principal results from the Women's Health Initiative randomized controlled trial." *JAMA,* 2002; 288 (3): 321–33.

Simon, J. A., et al. "One-year long-term safety extension study of ospemifene for the treatment of vulvar and vaginal atrophy in postmenopausal women with a uterus." *Menopause,* 2013 Apr; 20 (4): 418–27.

Soe, L. H., et al. "Ospemifene for the treatment of dyspareunia associated with vulvar and vaginal atrophy: Potential benefits in bone and breast." *Int J Womens Health,* 2013 Sep 25; 5: 605–11.

Index

About the Author

BARB DEHN, R.N., M.S., N.P., is a women's health nurse practitioner in private practice and a much sought-after television commentator on health issues. She earned a master's degree from the University of California, San Francisco, and a bachelor of science degree from Boston College. Barb is certified as a menopause practitioner by the North American Menopause Society and is a Fellow in the American Academy of Nurse Practitioners.

In addition to national appearances on CNN, NBC, and CBS, Nurse Barb, as she is known, took the extraordinary leap of bringing her blog, *Nurse Barb's Daily Dose,* to national television via ABC television. She is the award-winning author of a series of guides to women's health, including *Your Personal Guide to Menopause* and *Your Personal Guide to Pregnancy,* which are used by millions of women in the United States.

Barb lives in the San Francisco Bay area with her husband and son.